Seasoned with Lavender

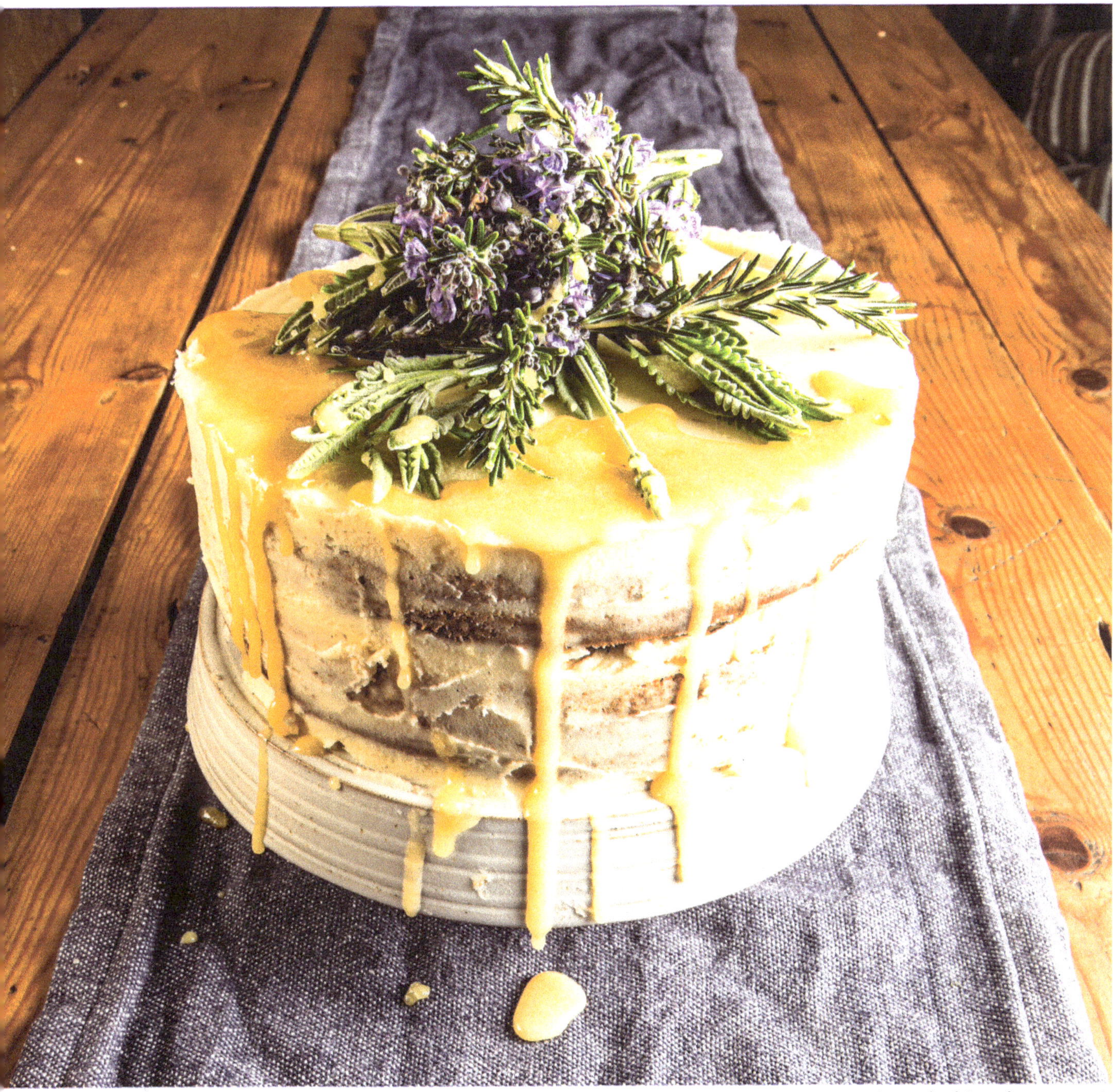

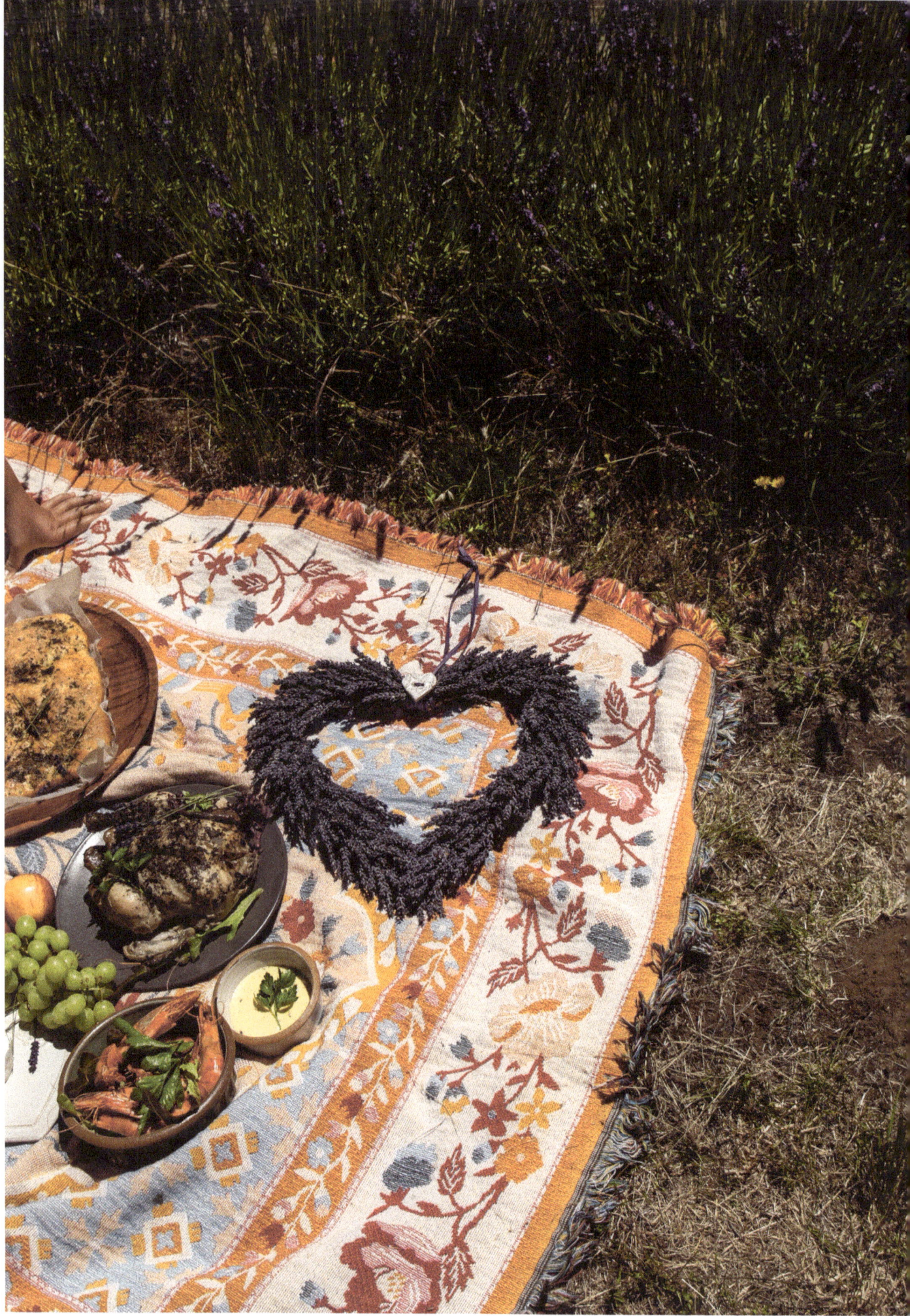

Acknowledgements

Thank you to my workshop participants and guests at Little Norfolk Bay Bistro and Chalets, who taste all the recipes and inspire me to create new dishes.

Thanks to my family, my husband Brendan and children Maggie, Stephanie and Oscar for their support and modelling in the photos.

Thanks to Kylie Berry Design for the beautiful design and support with the creation of this book.

Thanks to my mum Bernadette Heaney and daughter Maggie Emmett for editing.

Thanks to Lisa Britzman's from Campo De Flori farm for providing a beautiful place for our photos in the lavender farm.

And a big thanks to the sponsors and recipe contributors that have made this book possible and have been so helpful, encouraging and enthusiastic to work with on this project:

Lisa Britzman, Campo de Flori

Kim Weston, Bridestowe Estate

Daniel, Rannoch Quail Tasmania

Clare Dean, Port Arthur Lavender Farm

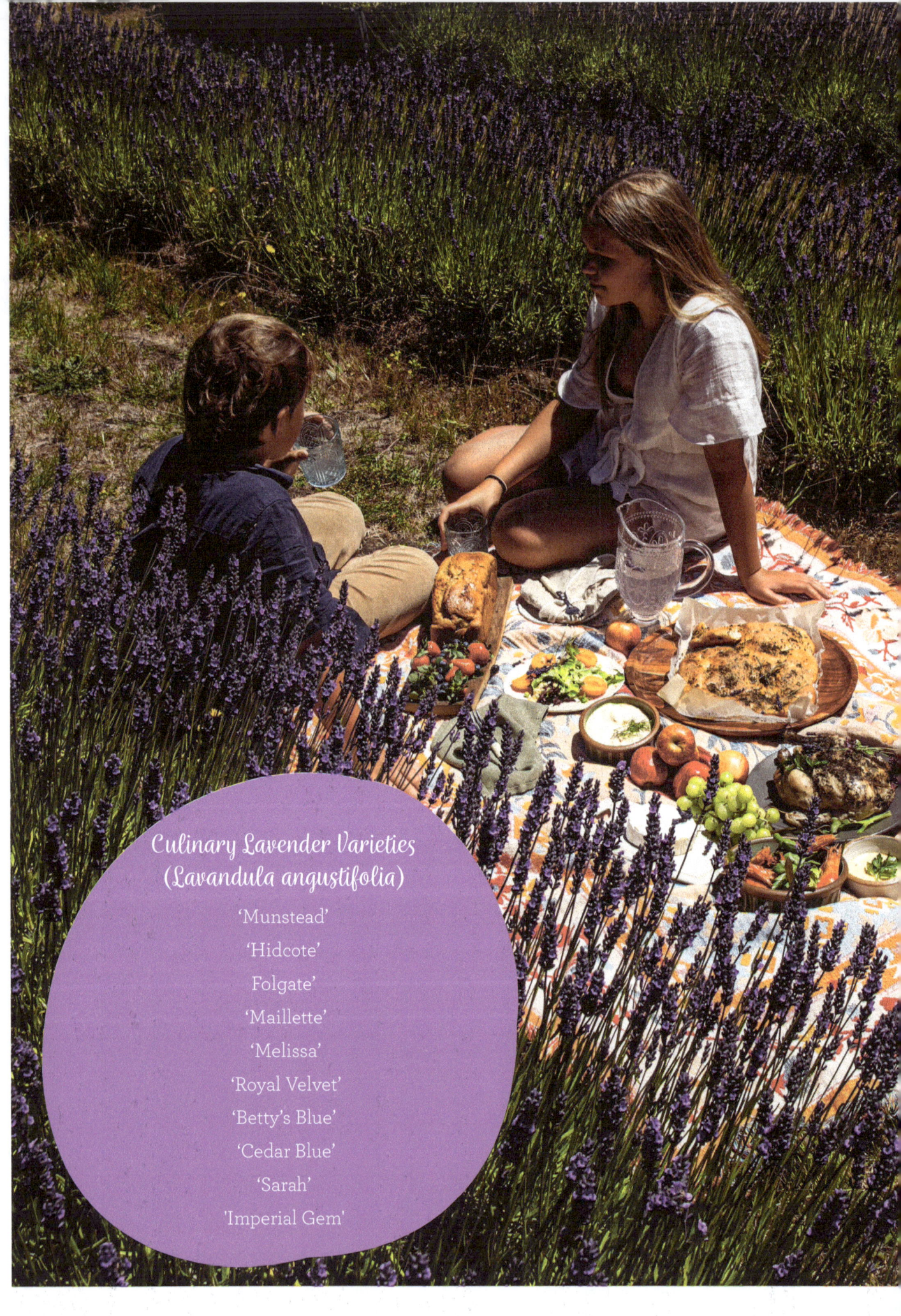

Culinary Lavender Varieties
(Lavandula angustifolia)

'Munstead'

'Hidcote'

'Folgate'

'Maillette'

'Melissa'

'Royal Velvet'

'Betty's Blue'

'Cedar Blue'

'Sarah'

'Imperial Gem'

Introduction

I first created the lavender and blueberry butter sauce in this book back in 2000, working as a chef de partie on Bedarra Island. But it wasn't until around 20 years later, whilst Chief Judge at the Hobart Fine Food Awards, that lavender truly took hold in my kitchen. That year, a culinary lavender from Campo de Flori caught my eye—beautifully grown, clean, and perfectly balanced. It completely changed the way I thought about lavender in food.

Until then, I'd filed lavender away in my mind alongside soaps, essential oils, and the little sachets Mum received every Mother's Day.

This was different the dried flowers had depth, complexity and subtlety.

I started with infused cream and desserts then moved into savoury territory: slow-cooked lamb, roast pumpkin, even fish. I discovered that, just like any strong herb, a little goes a long way. But when used with care, it adds something truly special, and to my surprise, it pairs brilliantly with seafood.

My passion has always been cooking with real food—fresh, seasonal ingredients prepared simply at home. I believe that's something worth holding onto in a world that endorses replacing the kitchen with plastic-wrapped, factory-made meals. Cooking from scratch isn't just healthier; it's more rewarding, more connected, and infinitely more delicious.

This book brings together those discoveries—recipes tested in my own kitchen, built around produce from the garden, the market, or the sea. Some are quick and easy, others more elaborate, but all show how culinary lavender can shine in everyday cooking.

If you're new to it, this is the perfect place to start.

Why Cook with Lavender?

There's something special about using ingredients straight from the garden or a local grower. Culinary lavender— those small purple buds— aren't just pretty. It has a unique flavour and a long history of being used for both food and natural remedies.

We now know that cooking with real, unprocessed ingredients is one of the best things for our health. If buying a bunch of culinary lavender gets you into the kitchen, thinking creatively and cooking from scratch, that's already a win.

Lavender, when used well, can really lift a dish. It's floral but not soapy, subtle but noticeable. It works beautifully with honey, lemon, lamb, seafood, chocolate, and soft cheeses—adding something a little different.

Beyond flavour, lavender has traditionally been used to support sleep, calm nerves, ease stress, and much more. Some of these benefits are backed by research, others come from generations of use. Either way, it's a herb known for its calming, soothing qualities. Researching the historical uses of lavender in health is fascinating. I particularly enjoyed reading about the 'four thieves' and lavender usage in ancient Roman times where it's benefits for brain health were recognised.

So whether cooking for flavour, wellness, or just for the joy of it, lavender is a lovely ingredient to try. If it brings you into the kitchen, helps you slow down, and makes food feel a bit more special—then that's more than enough of a reason.

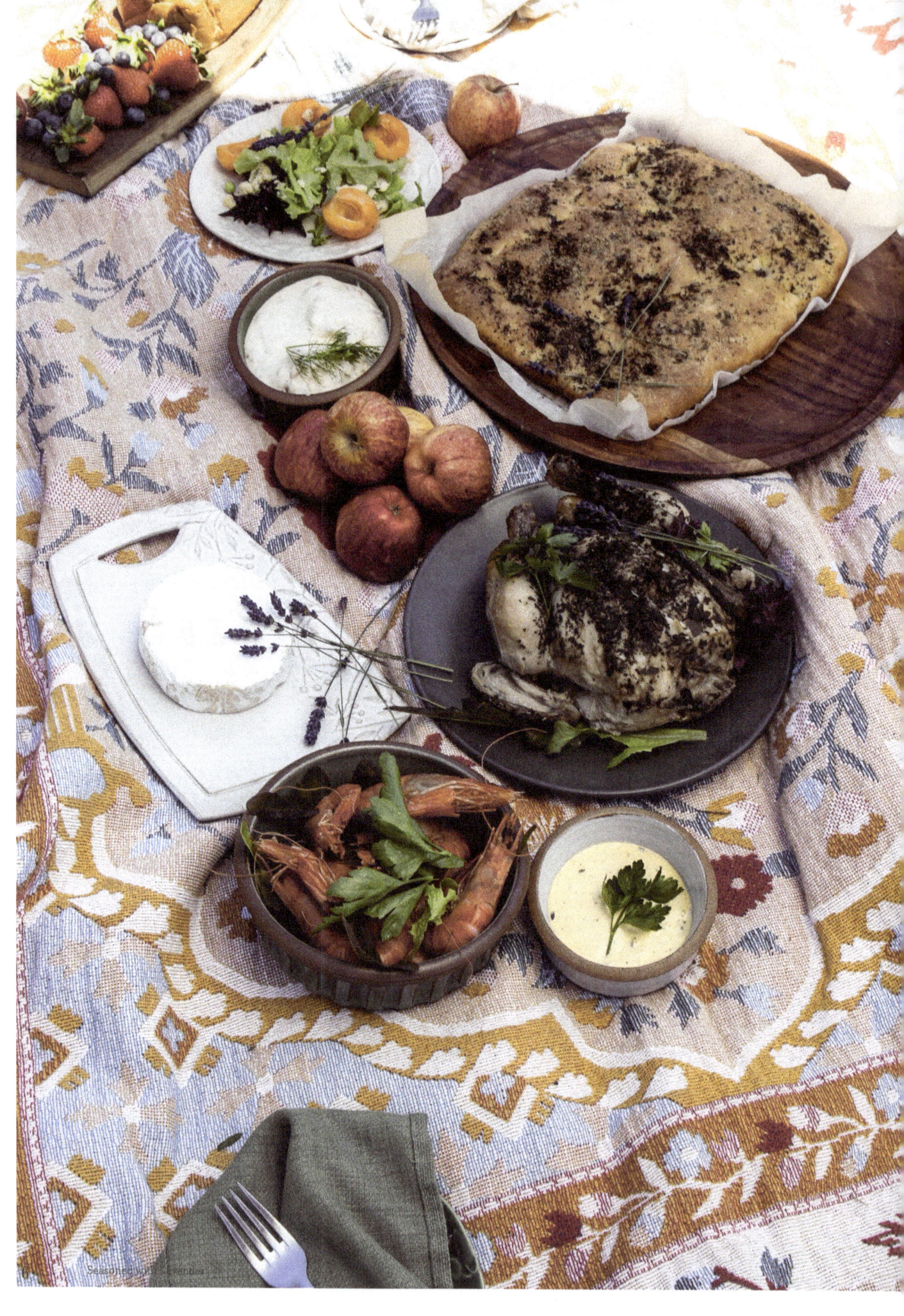

How to Cook with Lavender

Culinary lavender is delicate, fragrant, and best used with a light hand, a little goes a long way. When used thoughtfully, it brings a soft floral note to both sweet and savoury dishes.

Lavender has been used in food and medicine for thousands of years. Ancient civilisations—such as the Egyptians, Greeks, and Romans—valued lavender for its fragrance, therapeutic properties, and culinary potential. While more often used for bathing, perfuming, and preserving, it was also infused into oils, wines, and honey. In medieval kitchens and monasteries, it began appearing in herbal blends and sweets. Today, it's enjoying a resurgence in modern kitchens around the world, celebrated for both its unique flavour and wellness benefits.

While not poisonous, not all lavender is edible. The best variety for cooking is Lavandula angustifolia (often called English lavender). It has a softer, sweeter flavour than other types like Lavandula stoechas or Lavandula dentata, which can be too strong. Look for lavender specifically labelled for culinary use, or grow your own.

Most people cook with the dried or fresh buds, but the slender, silvery-green leaves are also edible. They carry a more herbaceous, slightly resinous note—milder than rosemary but beautifully aromatic.

The flowers are ideal for:

- Baking cakes and biscuits
- Infusions of milk, honey, vinegar or simple syrup
- Garnishes and dessert decoration

The leaves can be:

- Finely chopped and added to savoury dishes for example roast lamb.
- Steeped into oils or broths
- Dried and mixed with other herbs like rosemary, thyme, or sage

Lavender can easily overwhelm a dish if overused. Think of it as a seasoning, much like rosemary or mint. Start small—especially with dried culinary lavender, which has a more concentrated flavour. The essential oil is best reserved for desserts like a cheese cake when you want a punch of flavour.

Tips for use:

- Dry vs Fresh: Dried is stronger. If a recipe calls for dried culinary lavender and you're using fresh, double the amount.
- Infusions: Steep lavender in warm liquids—milk, cream, honey, vinegar—then strain before using.
- Pairings: Lavender works especially well with lemon, honey, berries, vanilla, white chocolate, lamb, seafood, poultry, goat cheese, and root vegetables.

Lavender is often blended with other herbs, especially in the French classic Herbes de Provence. Try mixing it with thyme, rosemary, and marjoram for a fragrant rub or sprinkle. I like a Tasmanina bush version with salt bush, native thyme, native oregano, lemon myrtle and some pepperberries.

Dry the buds and leaves in a dark, well-ventilated spot, and store them in airtight jars away from sunlight. Use within a year for best flavour.

Lavender works well as a mild background flavour, not the main act. When balanced well, it lifts a dish with a subtle floral brightness.

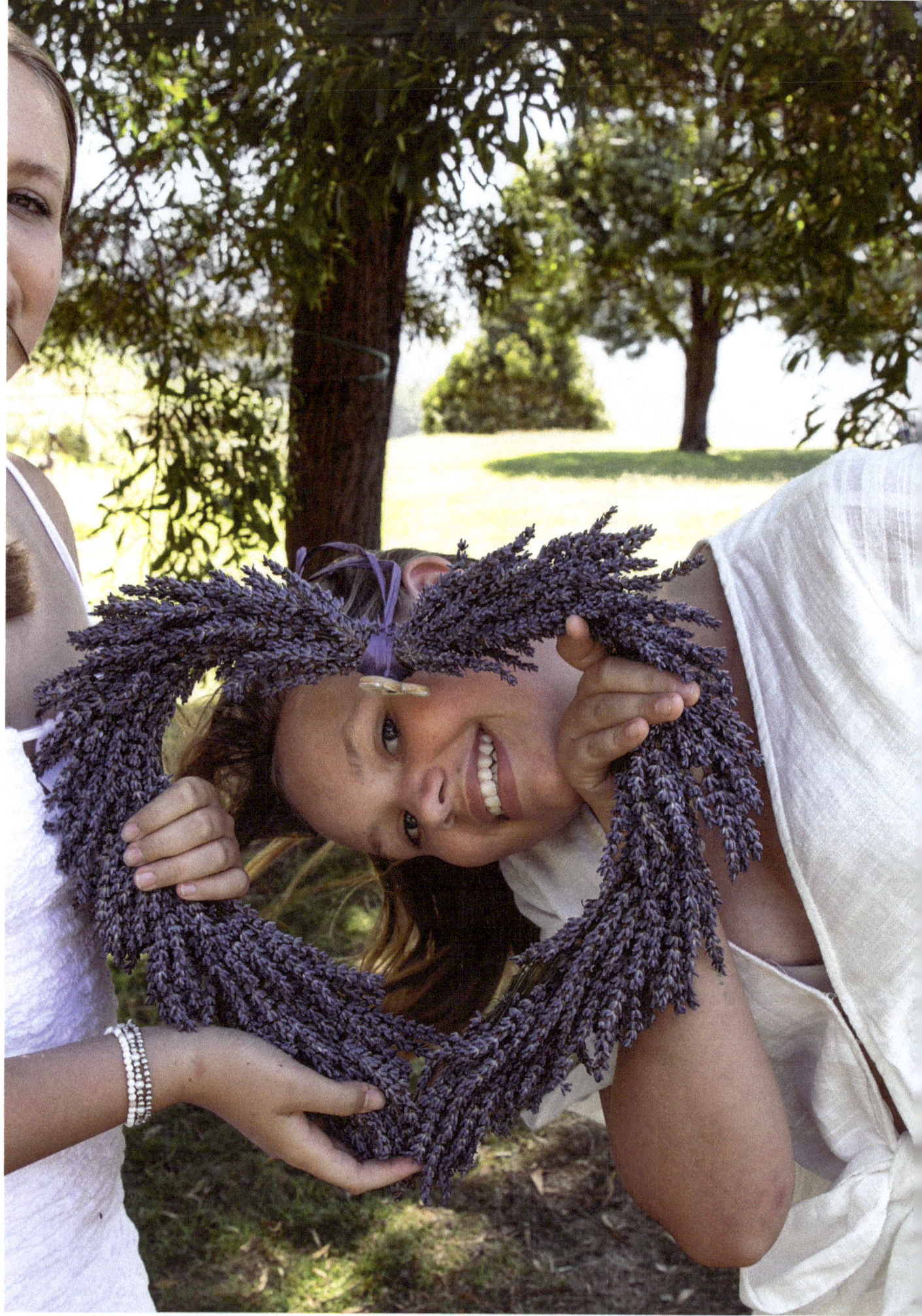

Mystical Properties of Lavender

I would prefer to use lavender in cleaning products in my home simply to avoid harsh chemicals but for some fun lets look at the magical properties of lavender:

Common Uses:

Protection:

- Burn dried lavender as incense to cleanse a space of negative energies.
- Add it to protective sachets or spell jars to ward off evil.

Love and Attraction:

- Use in love spells or charm bags to attract romance or deepen emotional bonds.
- Sprinkle a bit of lavender oil or dried flowers on your bed or pillow for sensuality and affection.

Calming and Sleep Magic:

- Place lavender under your pillow or in a dream sachet to prevent nightmares and encourage peaceful sleep.
- Use it in bath rituals to relieve stress and promote tranquility.

Purification and Cleansing:

- Add to ritual baths or floor washes to spiritually cleanse yourself or your home.
- Use in smoke cleansing with sage to purify objects or spaces.
- Hang a small bundle of lavender above your front door for harmony.
- Self-Love Ritual: Infuse a candle with lavender oil and meditate with affirmations.
- Protection Jar: Combine lavender, rosemary and salt in a small jar for a portable ward.

Potato, Leek and Ham Soup with Herbs de Provence

MAKES A FEW FAMILY BATCHES

This soup is a great use for the leftover ham bone. A batch of Herbs de Provence made up from dried or fresh herbs is always a handy addition to any kitchen or simply purchase from Bridestowe Estate. This aromatic herb mix can be added to roast chicken, lamb, soups, grilled meats and more.

FOR THE STOCK

one meaty ham bone

1 onion

1 leek

1 large carrot

2 sticks celery

20 peppercorns

few sprigs parsley

few sprigs thyme

6 bay leaves

TO MAKE THE SOUP

2 kilos potatoes

1 carrot

1 leek

2 onions

5 cloves garlic

1 tablespoon butter

200ml cream

1-2 tablespoons Herbs de Provence (made from lavender, thyme, oregano, basil, rosemary, marajoram)

To make your ham stock: Place the ham bone into a slow cooker or a large stovetop pot. Add diced onion, celery, leek and carrot. (At home, I collect offcuts of these while cooking and keep a bag in the freezer—when it's time to make stock, I just grab a few handfuls.). Add a few peppercorns, sprigs of parsley, bay leaves and thyme and just enough water to cover the ingredients. The key to a really tasty, aromatic stock is not to add too much water—keep it concentrated. Simmer gently on the stovetop for a few hours, until the meat is falling off the bone. In a slow cooker, cook on high for around 5 hours, though times can vary depending on your slow cooker.

To prepare the soup: Peel and dice onion, carrot, leek, and garlic. Sauté gently in a large heavy-based pot with a generous lump of butter until softened. Add the ham stock, making sure to remove all the ham from the bone and return it to the pot. Stir in a few tablespoons of Herbes de Provence. Cook until the potatoes are soft and tender. Blend the soup until smooth, then season with salt and pepper to taste. Finish with a swirl of cream before serving.

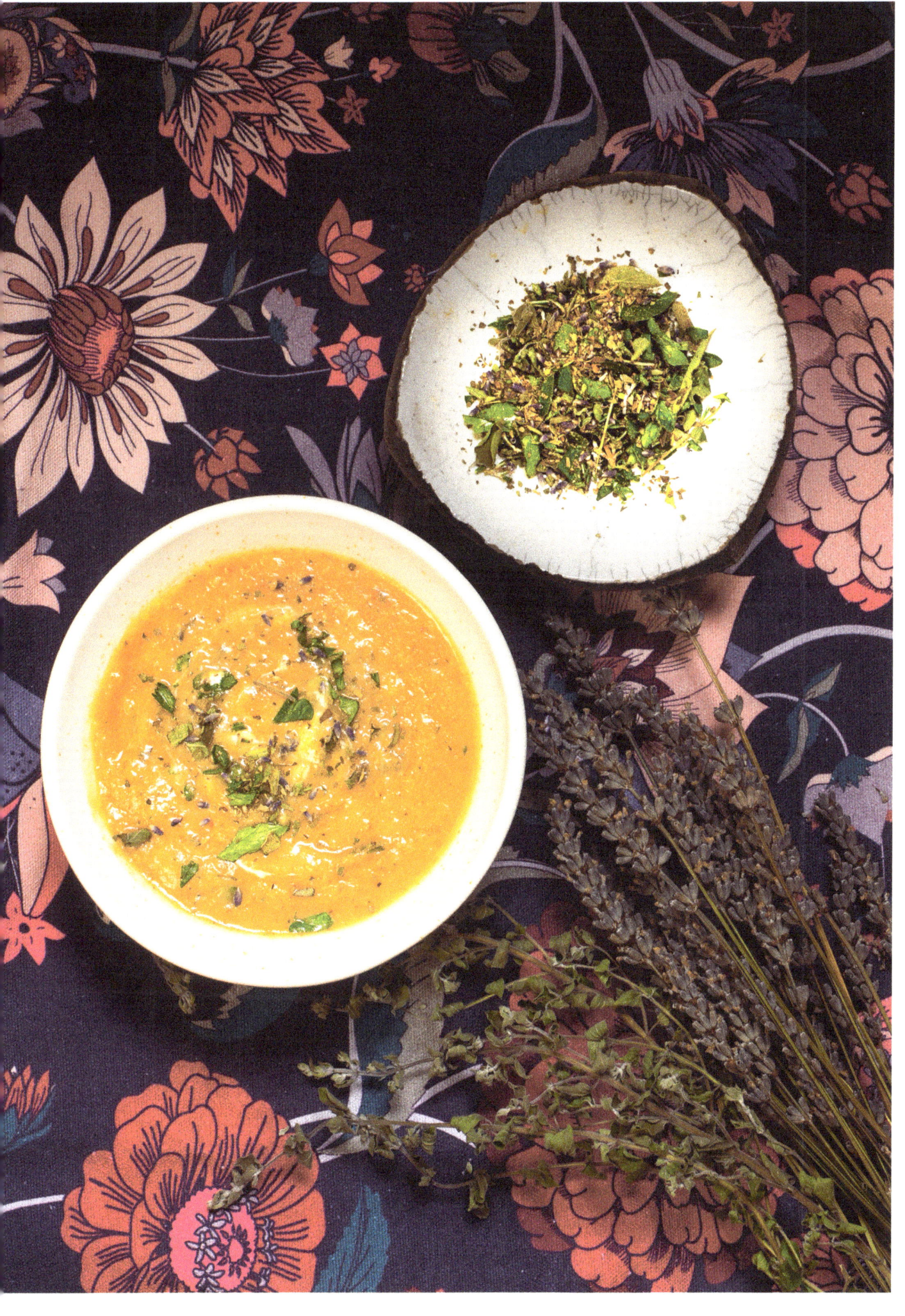

Buttermilk Fried Rannoch Quail

SERVES 4 FOR AN ENTREE

If you make your own butter you are always looking for a use for the left over butter milk. Substitute with regular milk if you need. We are using one large quail as an entree for this dish, like we serve in the bistro, however many people find a large quail enough for a main course or lunch with a bigger salad. Or you can use the quail breast.

4 Rannoch Quail Tasmania boned quails or quail breast meat

extra virgin olive oil for cooking

1 cup buttermilk

1 teaspoon dijon mustard

½ teaspoon black pepper

½ teaspoon tarragon

½ teaspoon thyme

½ teaspoon dried culinary lavender

½ teaspoon salt

100 grams plain flour

Mix together salt, pepper, lavender, tarragon, thyme, mustard, and milk. Add the quail and marinate overnight in the fridge.

When you're ready to cook, heat oil for frying—either shallow or deep, depending on your equipment and preference. For the crispiest, most evenly cooked result, deep frying is best. Heat the oil to 170°C.

Remove each quail from the marinade, letting any excess drip off. Coat thoroughly in plain flour, then carefully lower into the hot oil. Fry until golden brown and just cooked through—this will take about 6 minutes in a deep fryer. You may want to check the thickest part of the breast with a knife to ensure it's cooked through.

Alternatively, you can pan-fry the floured quail in a small amount of oil in a large, heavy-based pan—about 5 minutes on each side or until crisp and cooked through.

Drain on paper towel to remove any excess oil and serve hot with your favourite chutney and a fresh garden salad.

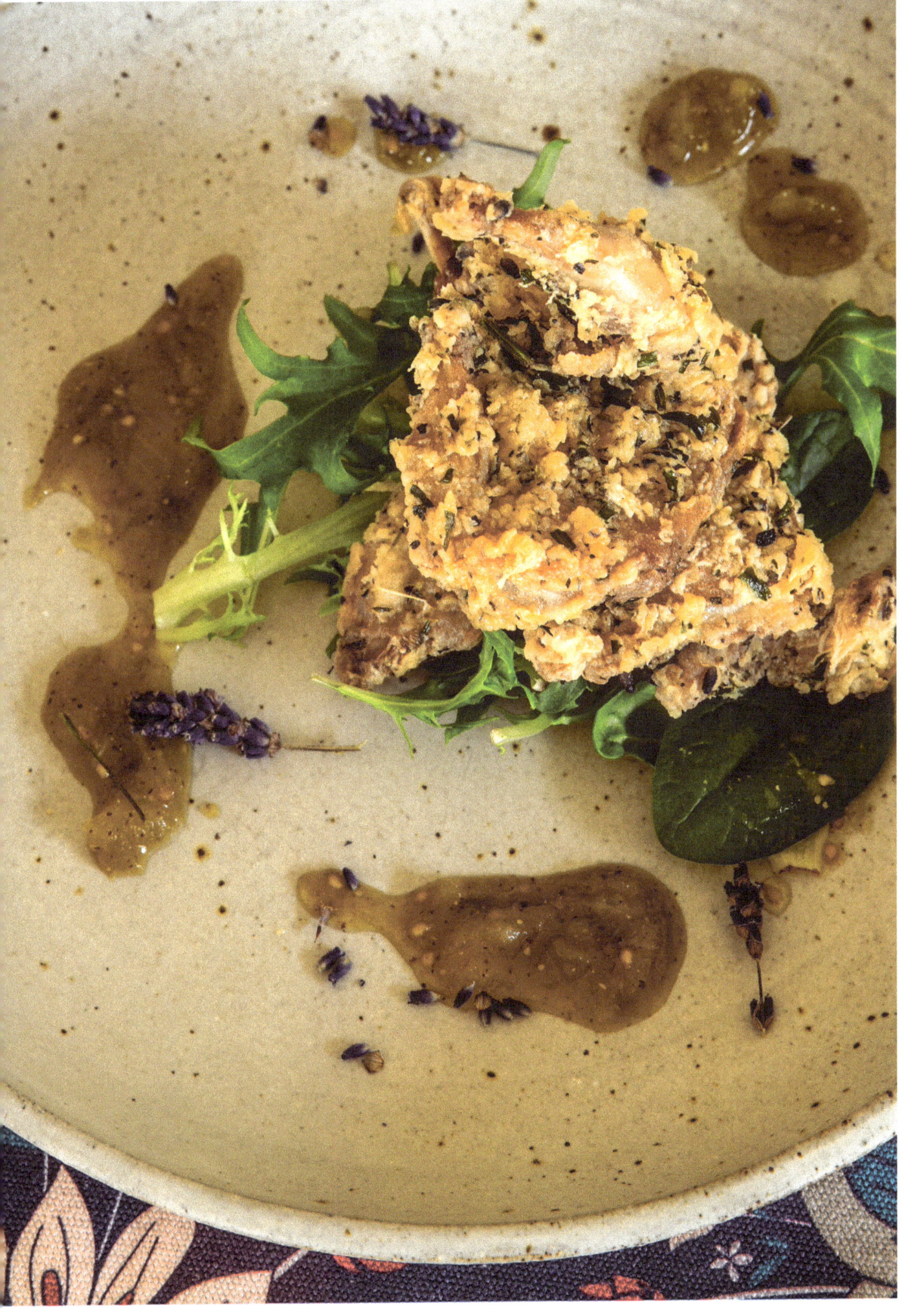

Duck with Mulberry and Lavender Relish and Apple Slaw

SERVES 6

We are lucky in the bistro to have an amazing supply of Mulberries from a neighbour so when we have made enough jam, we make this relish that goes well with many savoury dishes.

6 duck marylands

extra virgin olive oil

SLAW

1 tablespoon apple cider vinegar

2 tablespoons robust extra virgin olive oil

1 green apple

¼ red cabbage

2 carrots

3 spring onion

sea salt

white pepper

MULBERRY AND LAVENDER RELISH

1 brown onion

1 teaspoon oil

2 cloves garlic

½ teaspoon ginger

2 cups mulberries

50ml red wine vinegar

½ cup brown sugar

1 teaspoon culinary lavender

½ cracked pepper

good pinch salt

Heat the oven to 120°C

In a large heavy based pan seal the duck marylands over a medium high heat, making sure the skin sides gets an extra minute for a crispy skin. Place the maryland in a baking dish. The trick here is to find a dish where they fit snuggly into when laid out flat - so you won't need as much oil to cover them.

Cover the marylands with oil then cover the dish with foil and cook in a 120°C oven for around 4 hours until the meat is tender and falling from the bone. The leftover oil can be stored in the fridge to use in the next few days for your cooking.

To make the slaw, finely slice or grate the apple, carrot, cabbage, spring onion and mix with the vinegar and oil, season well with the salt and pepper.

To make the relish, finely slice the onion, garlic and ginger and sauté in a heavy based pan with the oil. Add the brown sugar, berries and vinegar and continue to cook until the relish reduces into a thick sauce. This will take around 30 minutes on a low heat. Add the lavender towards the end of the cooking and season well with salt and pepper.

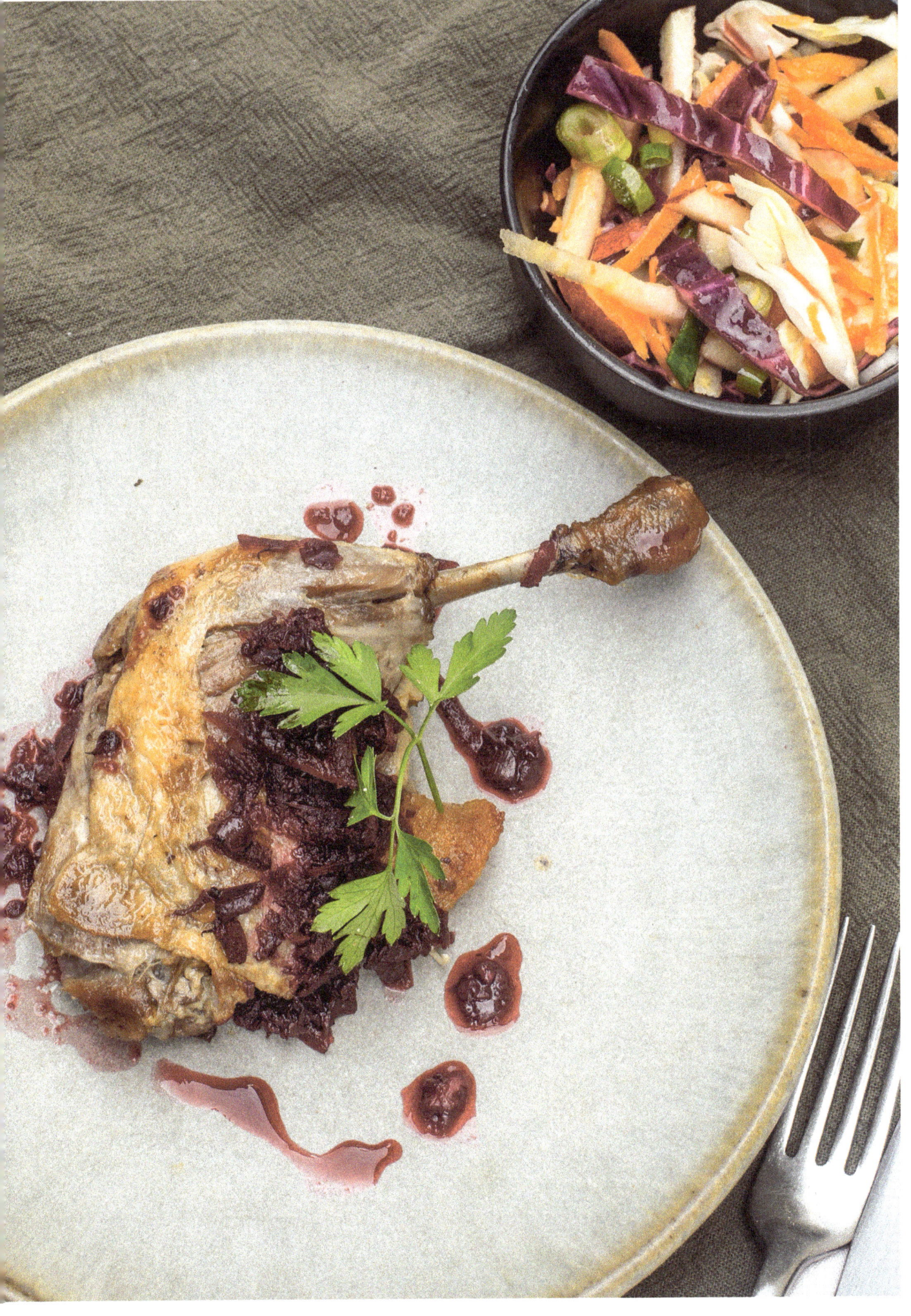

Lavender and Blueberry Pancakes

SERVES 6

These pancakes are perfect for a special breakfast.

2 cups self-raising flour

¼ cup castor sugar

2 eggs

2 cups of milk

1 teaspoon vanilla essence

1 tablespoon butter

1 teaspoon dried culinary lavender

1 cup blueberries

TO SERVE

Fruit sauce or coulis, yogurt, ice-cream, cream or chocolate sauce

In a large mixing bowl add the flour, salt and sugar. Make a well in the centre and add the eggs and whisk. Next add the milk, lavender and vanilla essence, combine and then whisk until smooth.

Heat a large non-stick frying pan over a medium heat and add a small knob of butter and melt over pan. Add spoonfuls of batter to the pan and cook the pancakes for 2-3 minutes or until bubbles appear on the surface.

Flip and continue to cook for a few minutes until cooked through.

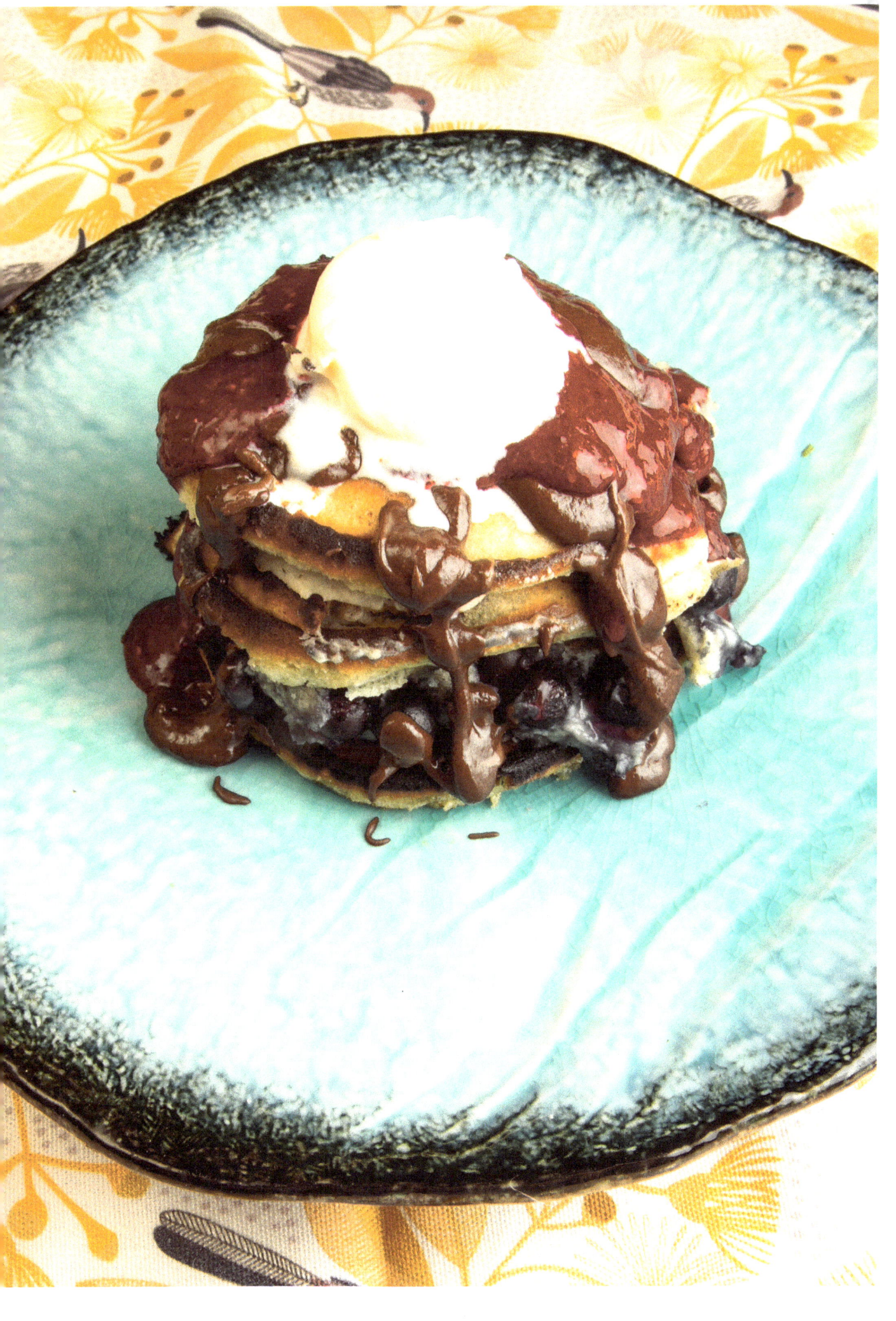

White Chocolate Lavender Cookies

MAKES 24 SMALL COOKIES

Lavender and white chocolate is a beautiful match, I have started very mildly with this recipe just one teaspoon of lavender but it can be increased to suit your taste.

125 grams butter
165 grams brown sugar
1 egg
1 teaspoon vanilla essence
1 teaspoon dried culinary lavender
150 grams plain flour
160 grams self-raising flour
200 grams white chocolate
150 grams macadamia nuts

Preheat oven to 175°C.

Line a baking tray with non-stick baking paper. Using a bowl or food processor, beat the butter and brown sugar until thick and creamy. Add egg, lavender and vanilla essence and continue to beat until well combined.

Fold in the plain flour and self-raising flour until just combined, then add the chopped white chocolate and macadamias to form a chunky mixture.

Place spoonfuls of the cookie mixture on the prepared tray and gently press down to flatten a little. Bake for 15-20 minutes or until golden brown. Remove from oven and set aside for a few minutes to cool slightly, then transfer to a wire rack to cool completely.

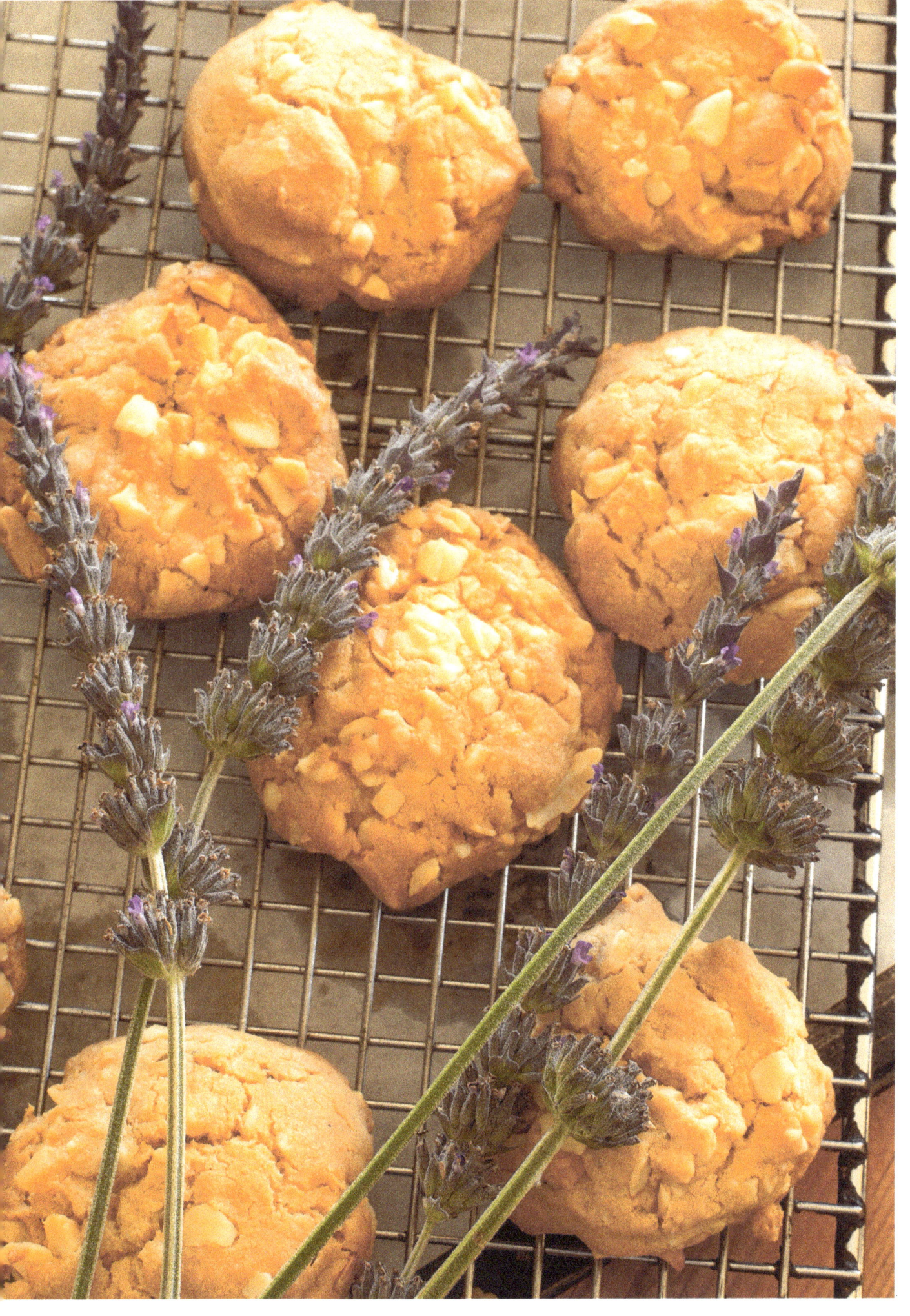

Rosemary, Garlic and Lavender Pull Apart Bread

SERVES 8

The easiset way to elavate what could be a boring dish like a simple pumkin soup is an amazing bread to serve with it, like this delicious pull apart bread.

BREAD DOUGH

500 grams plain or bakers flour

1 teaspoon yeast

1 teaspoon salt

1 teaspoon sugar

1 teaspoon bread improver

300ml - 320ml luke warm water

FOR THE BUTTER

4 cloves garlic

½ bunch fresh parsley

1 tablespoon fresh rosemary

2 teaspoons dry lavender

1 tablespoon extra virgin olive oil

½ teaspoon sea salt

¼ teaspoon cracked pepper

100 grams brie cheese

Knead all the bread ingredients together to create a smooth dough. I do this in the thermocooker with the knead function for 2 minutes. Alternatively mix by hand in a bowl and knead for around 10 minutes on a floured bench.

Place the dough in a bowl and cover and leave to rise in a warm spot for 30 minutes or until doubled in size.

To make the herb and garlic butter whip all ingredients together in the blender.

Heat the oven to 180°C.

Roll dough onto a floured board into large rectangle and spread herb butter over dough. If necessary, sprinkle dough with flour first to prevent butter from sliding off.

With a butter knife, cut 3-4cm wide strips. Fold each dough strip in half lengthways and place cut side up in a 26cm spring form tin until all the strips are pressed in together. Leave to rise in a warm spot for about 20 minutes until it is filling the tin well.

Bake for approximately 40-45 minutes.

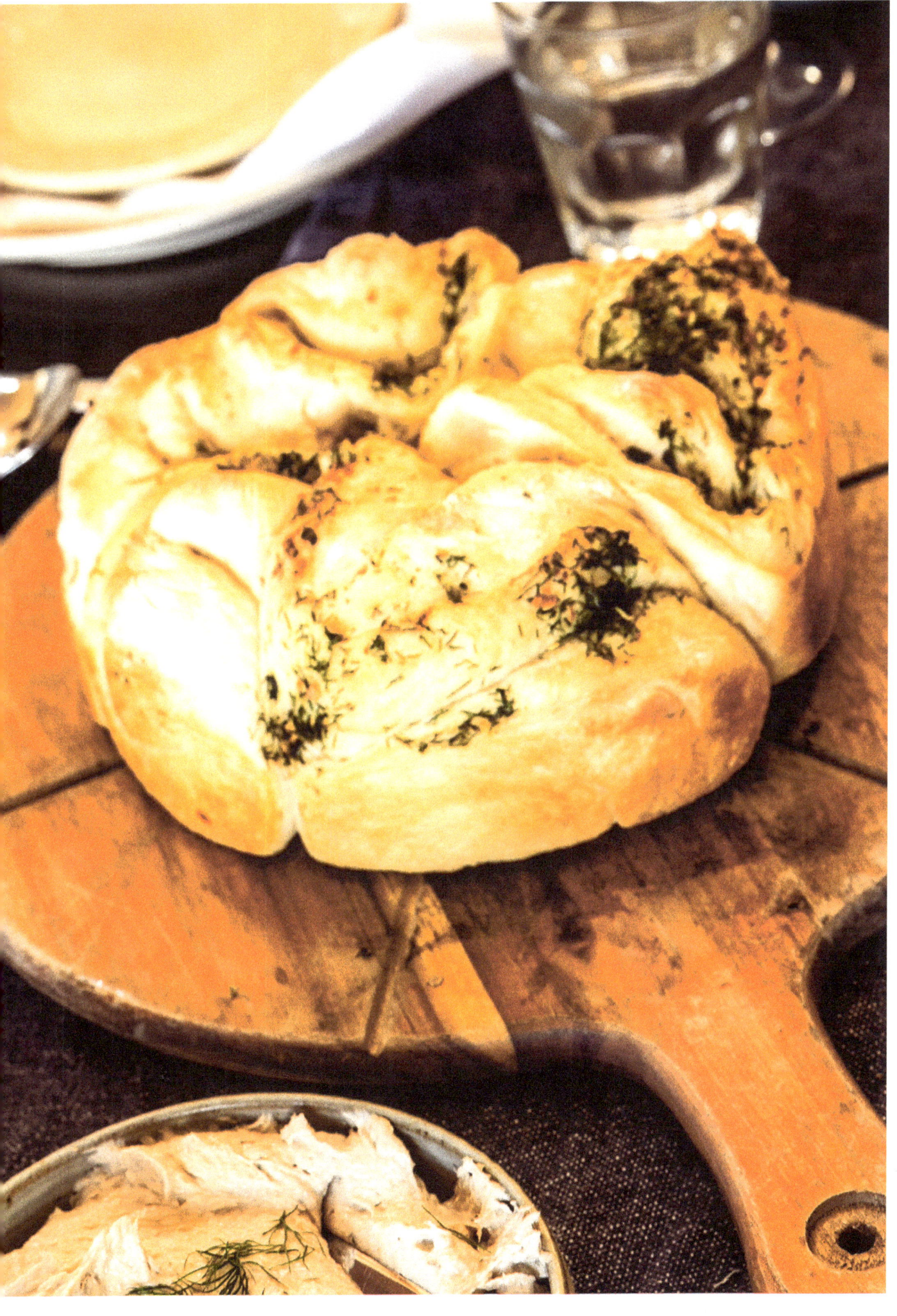

Goats Cheese and Lavender Beetroot Tart

SERVES 4

TART BASE

125 grams butter

1 2/3 cups plain flour

1 tablespoon water

TART FILLING

2 medium beetroot

2 bulbs garlic

1 tablespoon olive oil

half small brown onion

1 tablespoon basil leaves

1 teaspoon dried culinary lavender

100 grams goat cheese

2 tablespoons parmesan cheese

6 eggs

¾ cup cream

Preheat the oven to 180°C.

Grease a 20cm pie dish or tart tin.

To cook the vegetables for the tart, dice the beetroot into 1cm cubes and peel the garlic cloves. Tip beetroot and garlic into a baking tray, drizzle oil over to coat and roast in the oven for 18 minutes, or until soft and cooked through. Set aside to cool.

Meanwhile, use a food processor to make the pastry. Cut the butter into cubes, tip the flour into the processor, and pulse until the mixture resembles fine crumbs. With the motor running, add the water and process until the mixture forms a smooth dough, you may need to add a little extra water to help the mixture come together. Knead well on a floured bench, wrap in plastic wrap and set aside to rest for half an hour. Roll the pastry out to 5mm thick used to line the pie dish.

To make the tart filling, dice the onion and shred the basil leaves, chop the goat cheese and grate the Parmesan. In a large bowl, whisk together the eggs and cream until well combined, then stir through the onion, basil, lavender, cheeses, beetroot and garlic and mix well. Pour the filling into the tart base. Bake in the oven for 18 minutes, or until golden brown

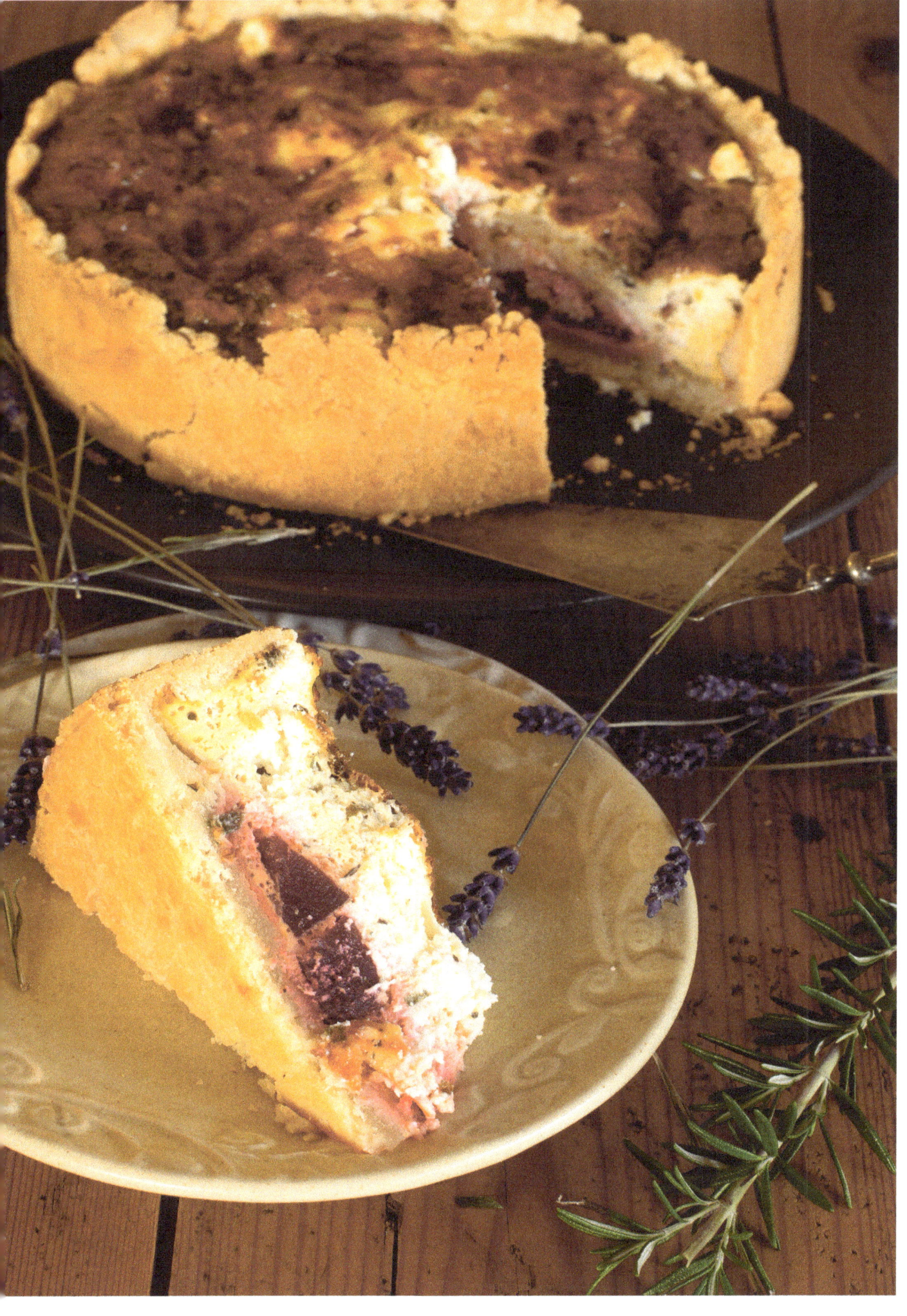

Pork Belly with Plum and Lavender

SERVES 4-6

1 large piece of pork belly - about 1 kilo

2 onions

10 plums

1 teaspoon ground fennel

1 teaspoon dried culinary lavender

4 sticks celery

6 cloves garlic

3 bay leaves

6 sprigs thyme

10 peppercorns

200ml white wine

1 litre stock (beef, veg, chicken)

TO SERVE

apple rissotto, apple slaw or mashed potatoes

Heat the oven to 160°C.

Seal the piece of pork in a large pan over a medium high heat so it is browned all over, lay the pork in a baking dish or you could use your slow cooker (adjust the cooking time).

Peel and slice the onion and slice the celery, remove the pip from the plums and chop into pieces, peel the garlic and add to the dish whole with the bay leaves, thyme, peppercorns, lavender, fennel and cover with the wine and stock.

Cover with kitchen foil and bake for 1.5-3 hours until cooked through. Size, thickness and the amount of fat is all going to affect the cooking time so it's best to put on early or even the day before.

To tell if it is cooked you should be able to poke it with a spoon and the meat will fall apart.

Purée the cooking liquid and plums to create a delicious sauce or serve in chunky rustic sityle. Serve with mashed potato or a tasty slaw such as an apple cider dressed apple, cabbage and carrot slaw.

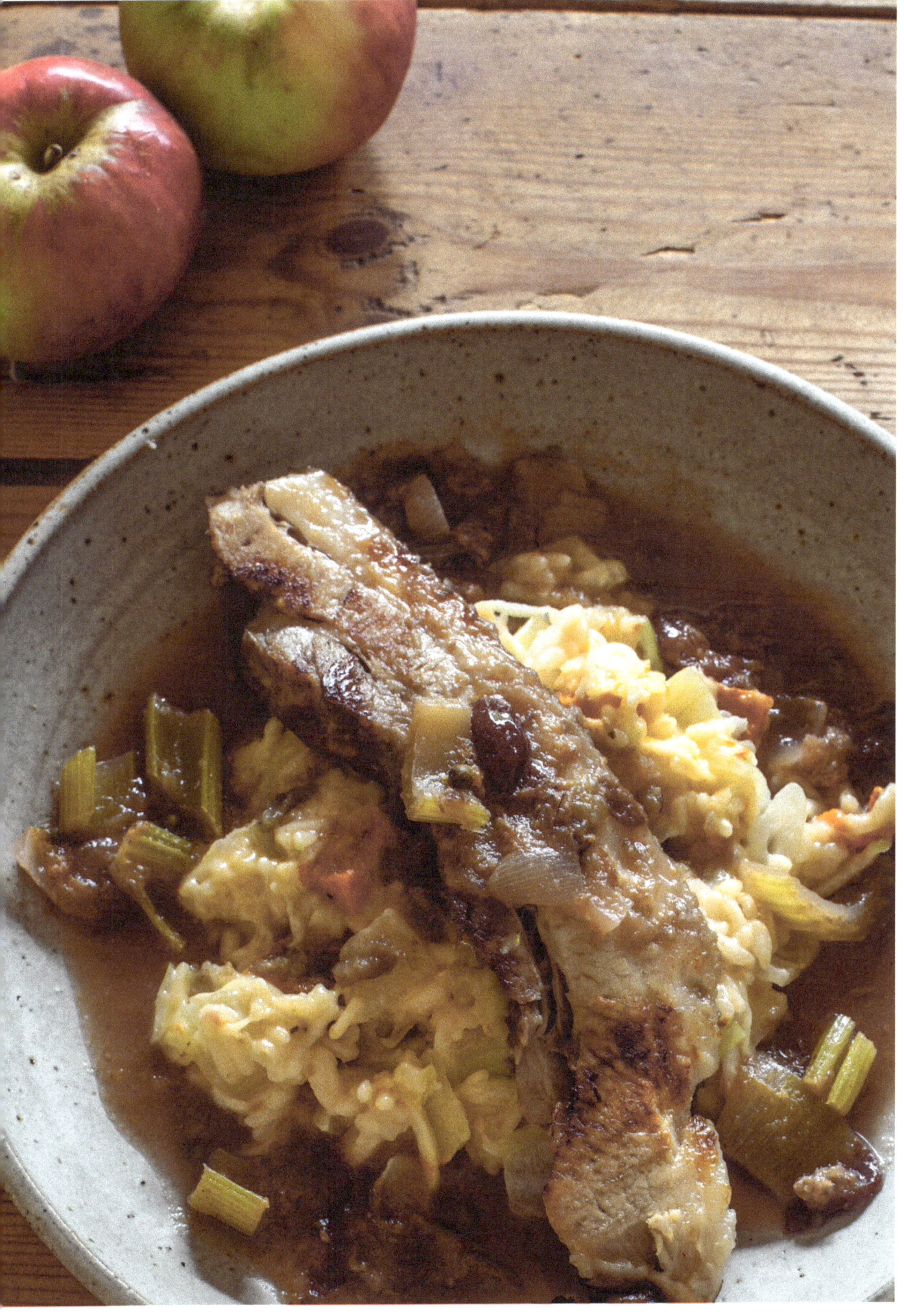

Sour Cherry, Verjuice and Lavender Jelly, Honey Custard Trifle

SERVES 4-6

Serve in a trifle dish or cute individual glasses.

500 grams lady finger biscuits or sponge cake

JELLY

200 grams sour cherries

400ml apple juice

100ml verjuice

2 tablespoons gelatine

2 teaspoons dried culinary lavender

CUSTARD

50 grams castor sugar

50 grams cornflour

500 grams full cream milk

4 eggs

2 tablespoons honey

Put half the apple juice in the blender with the cherries and blend until smooth. Bring the other half of the juice to a gentle boil in a pot on the stove with the verjuice and lavender, leave to infuse for at least 10 minutes. Add the cherry apple juice mix to the pot with the gelatine mix and bring gently back to a boil. Remove from the heat and add the geletine to dissolve. Strain. Pour the jelly into moulds, wine glasses or a triffle dish. Add the broken up biscuits or sponge and leave to set.

If you have a thermomix you'll know how to make custard in it (put it all in and cook for around 10 minutes). Or on the stove top bring the milk and honey to a gentle simmer. In a bowl crack the eggs and mix with the corn flour and sugar. Pour in the hot milk and mix well. Return to the stove and bring to a gentle simmer until cooked and thickened.

Pour the custard onto jelly and biscuits and leave to set in the refrigerator.

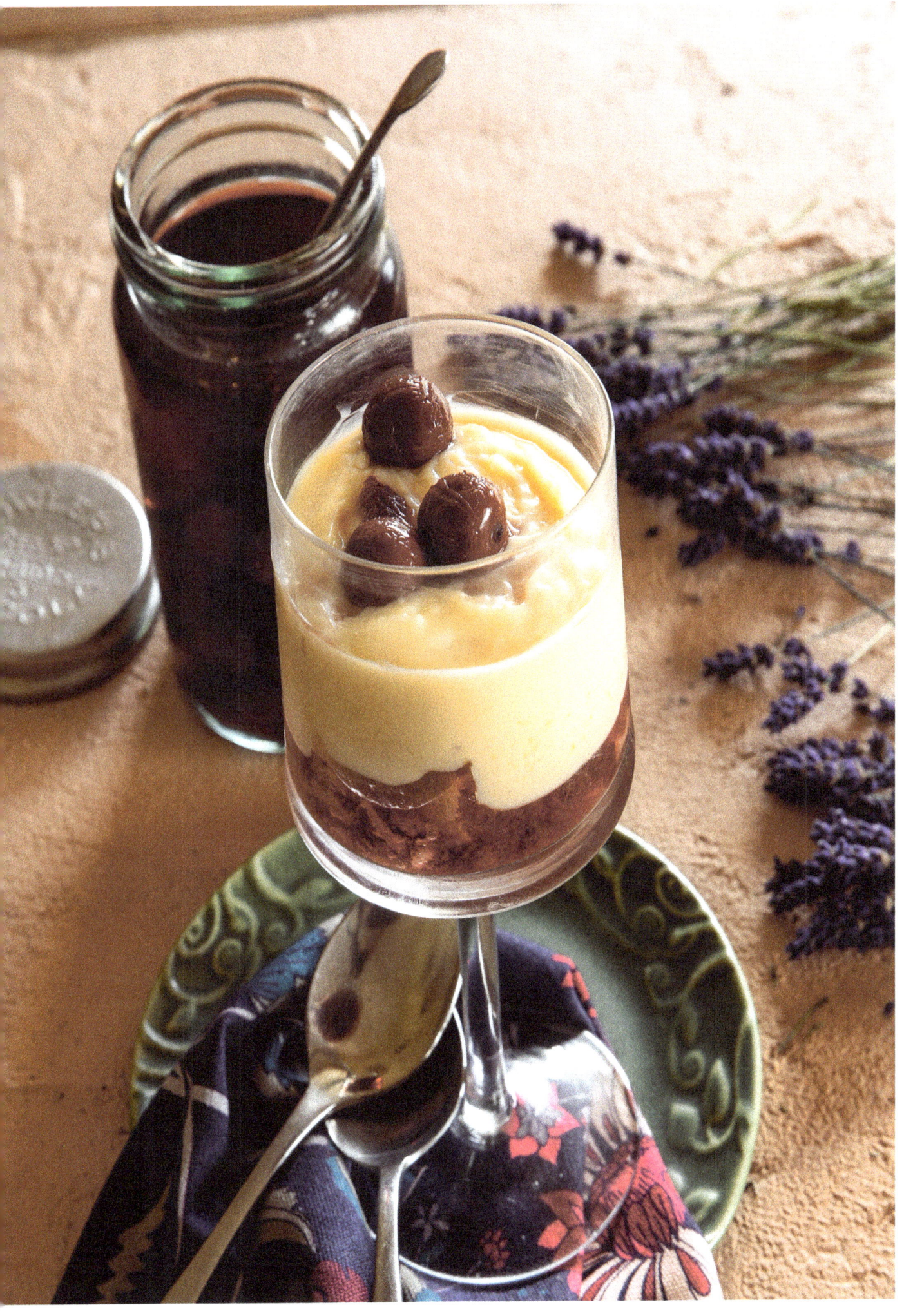

Venison Fillet Marinated with Pepperberry, Lavender Leaf and Rosemary with Spiced Quinces

SERVES 2

600 grams trimmed venison fillet

2 sprigs rosemary

2 sprigs fresh lavender leaf

1 tablespoon native pepperberries

dash of extra virgin olive oil

4 quinces

1 onion

1cm piece ginger

1 teaspoon ground cinnamon

1 teaspoon dried culinary lavender

½ teaspoon saffron threads

2 tablespoons brown sugar

2 teaspoons ground cumin

Begin by preparing the venison. Lightly crush the pepperberries and bruise the rosemary and lavender leaves to release their aromatic oils. Rub them into the fillet along with a dash of olive oil, coating the meat evenly. Leave it to marinate for at least two hours, or ideally overnight in the fridge, turning the meat once or twice during this time to let the flavours infuse.

To prepare the quince, peel and quarter them, removing the cores, then slice the onion and ginger. In a wide, heavy-based saucepan, heat a little olive oil over medium heat and slowly soften the onion and ginger until translucent and fragrant. Stir in the ground cinnamon, dried culinary lavender and cumin, cooking gently until the spices bloom. Add the brown sugar and allow it to melt and bubble slightly, then nestle the quinces into the pan. Pour in enough water so it comes up the sides of the fruit. Scatter over the saffron. Cover with a lid and let the quinces gently simmer on low heat for around an hour, turning occasionally until they soften and take on a rich amber colour in the spiced syrup.

When ready to serve, bring a cast iron pan or barbecue plate to high heat. Sear the venison on all sides until browned and cooked to medium rare – this should take about three to four minutes per side depending on the thickness of the fillet. Remove and rest the meat loosely covered for at least five minutes.

Slice the venison thickly across the grain and serve alongside the spiced quinces, spooning over some of the syrupy pan juices. A scattering of fresh herbs can finish the plate, served simply with mash or crusty sourdough.

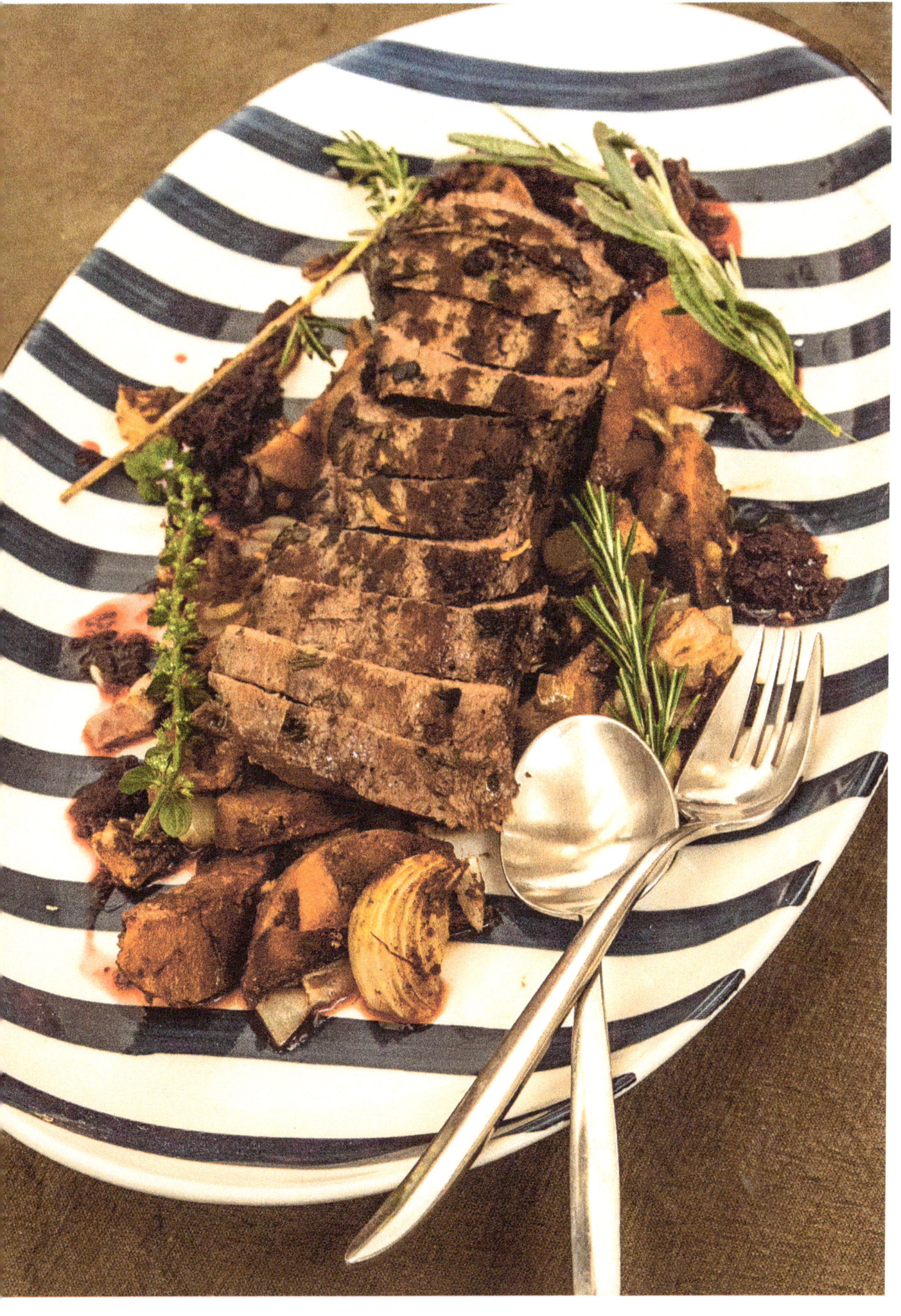

Porterhouse with Prawns in a Garlic and Herbs de Provence Sauce

SERVES 4

Beef and reef is an absolute classic and so delicious when it's made well! The essential ingredients are a good quality grilling steak (such as eye fillet, scotch fillet or porterhouse), real cream (not a white sauce) and fresh garlic (not out of a jar). Crayfish or scallops can be used instead of prawns. Follow this recipe and you can't go wrong.

4 porterhouse steaks

16 raw prawn cutlets

1 tablespoon extra virgin olive oil

½ small onion

2 cloves garlic

30ml white wine

200ml cream

sea salt and cracked pepper

2 tablespoons Herbs de Provence

To make the sauce, finely dice the onion and crush the garlic. Heat the oil in a heavy-based pan over low heat, and sauté the garlic and onion for three minutes, or until translucent. Add the prawns and deglaze the pan by pouring in the wine, then add the cream and simmer gently until the sauce thickens and the prawns are cooked, remove the prawns if the sauce needs a little more time to thicken. Add the provincail herbs to the sauce and season well with salt and pepper.

To cook your steak, preheat a grill pan (or the barbecue) to medium-high heat. Seal the steak on each side for 1 minute, reduce the heat to medium, and continue to cook to your liking. The time for cooking will depend on the thickness of your steak. One tip for cooking the steak, is that the fattier cuts will cook more quickly once the fat heats up – this is why a scotch fillet may take 10 minutes to get to medium, but only a couple more minutes to become well done. Use a meat thermometer if you are unsure, but take care not to prick the meat too many times, as you will lose the delicious juices. Wrap the steaks in foil for 5-10 minutes to rest before serving.

Serve the prawns and sauce on top of your rested steak, with a salad or veggies of your choice on the side.

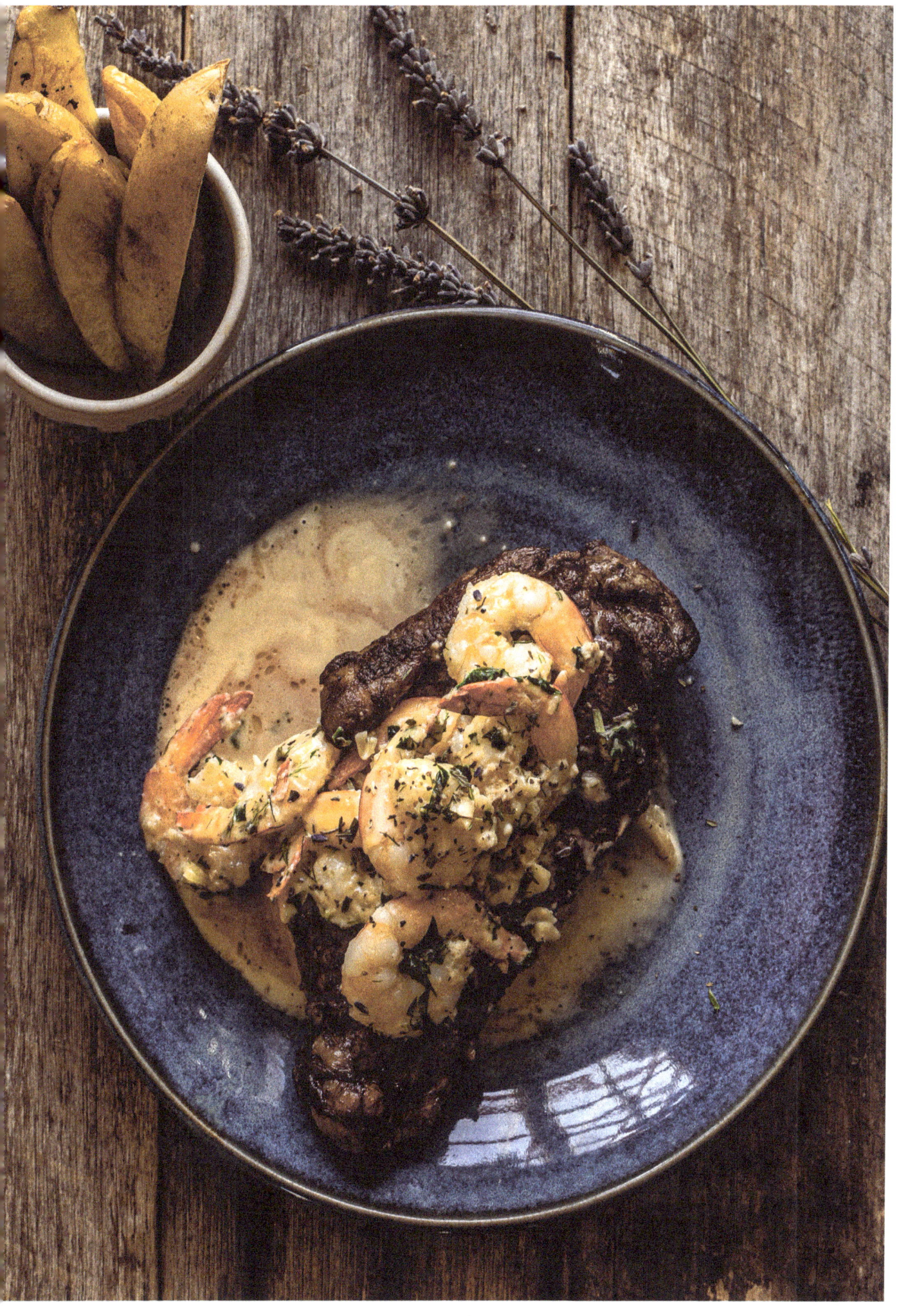

RECIPE BY BRIDESTOWE ESTATE LAVENDER

Duck Breast with Blueberry and Lavender Sauce

SERVES 2

2 duck breasts with skin on

4 tablespoons chopped shallots

2 tablespoons butter or extra virgin olive oil

100ml Pinot Noir

200ml chicken stock

2 generous tablespoons Bridestowe Gourmet Blueberry and Lavender Jam

Bridestowe Gourmet Pepper Plus to taste

Gently loosen some of the skin around the duck breast. Place duck breast skin side down on a hot nonstick frypan or barbeque plate. Cook gently until skin is very brown and fat has rendered.

This should take about 10 minutes. Turn breasts over and cook for 2-3 minutes or until medium rare. Avoid overcooking.

Meanwhile, in a small pan gently fry the chopped shallots until transparent. Add Pinot Noir and reduce to syrupy consistency.

Add chicken stock and reduce to one third volume.

Add Bridestowe Gourmet Blueberry and Lavender Jam and check for seasoning.

Serve over duck breasts accompanied by your favourite steamed vegetables and creamed potato

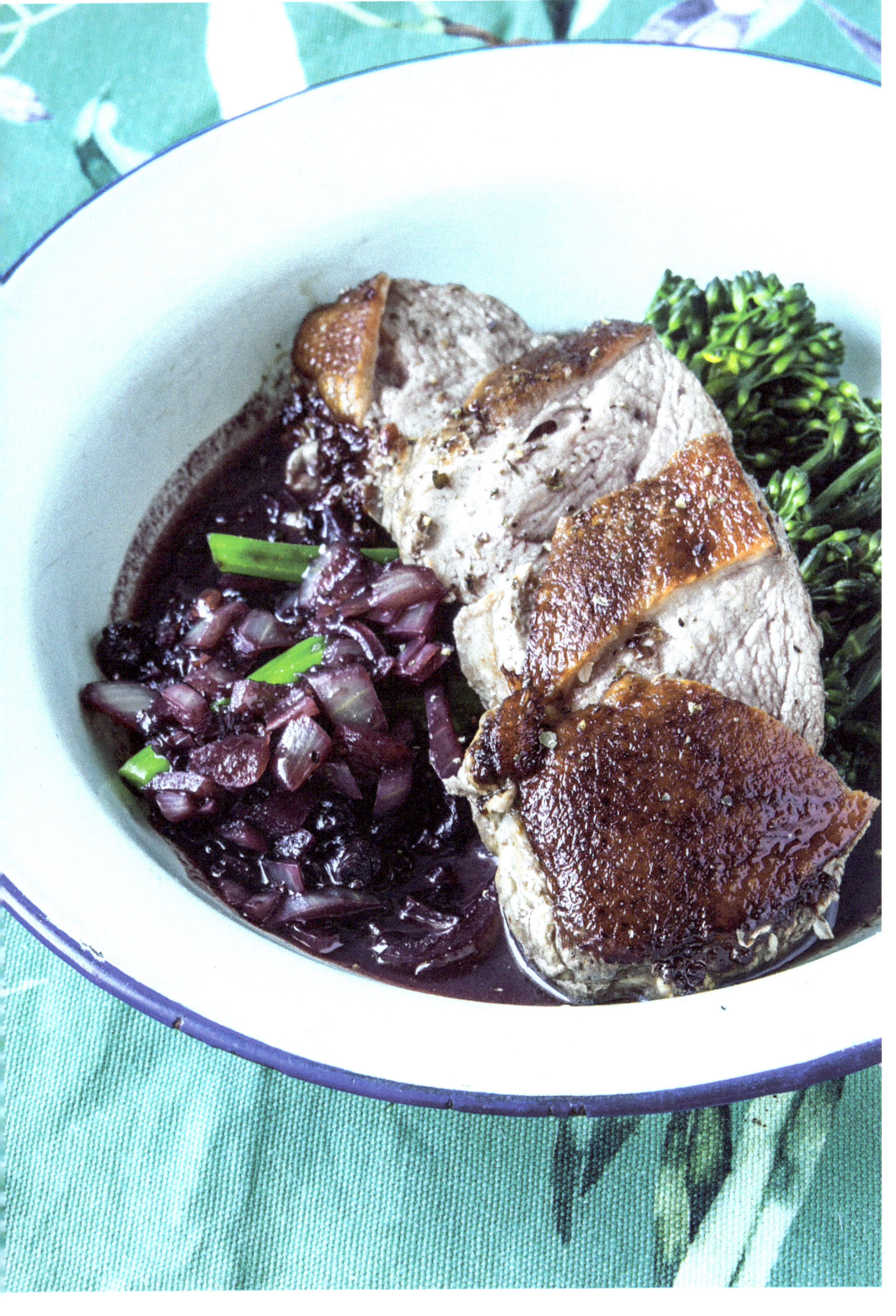

Lavender Mayonaise Prawn Cocktail

SERVES 4 FOR AN ENTREE OR LIGHT LUNCH

AIOLI

1 teaspoon dried culinary lavender

1 egg yolk

pinch sea salt

pinch white pepper

1 tablespoon apple cider vinegar

100ml delicate extra virgin olive oil

TO SERVE

½ lettuce

16 cooked prawns

To make the aioli, in the thermocooker or a blender or with a bowl whisk and strong fast-moving arm, add the yolk, vinegar, salt, pepper and lavender and blitz, pour the oil in a slow thin stream while continually blending or whisking to create a thick sauce.

Peel the prawns and wash and finely slice the lettuce and assemble into cute glasses or pots.

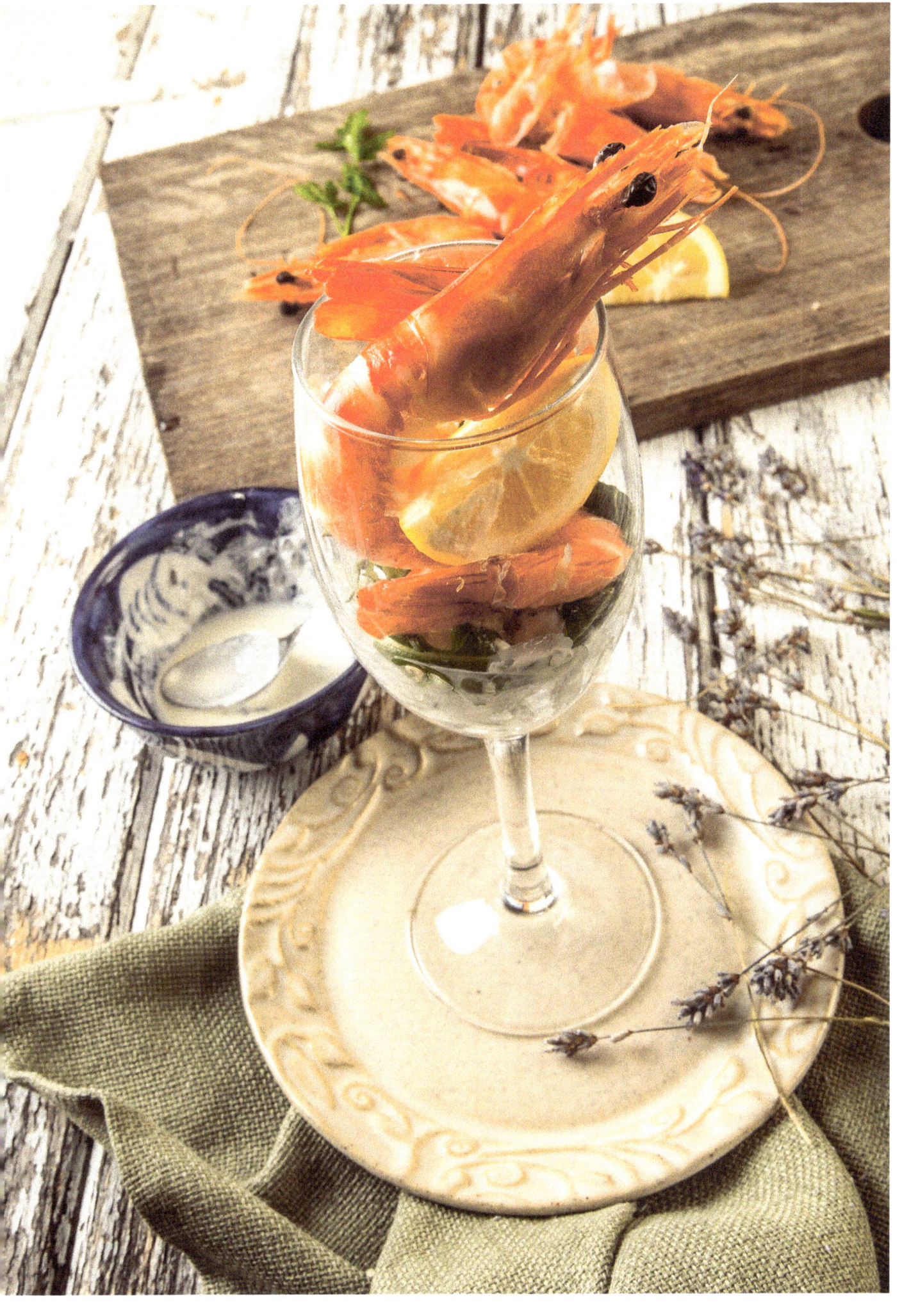

RECIPE BY BRIDESTOWE ESTATE LAVENDER

Watermelon Lavender Bubbly Cocktail

MAKES 1

30ml Bridestowe Lavender Gin
15ml freshly squeezed lemon juice
15ml Bridestowe Lavender Syrup
4 cubes watermelon approximately ¼ cup
90ml sparkling wine

In a shaker, muddle watermelon. Add ice and gin, syrup and lemon. Shake well.

Strain into flute or coupe glass and top with sparkling wine.

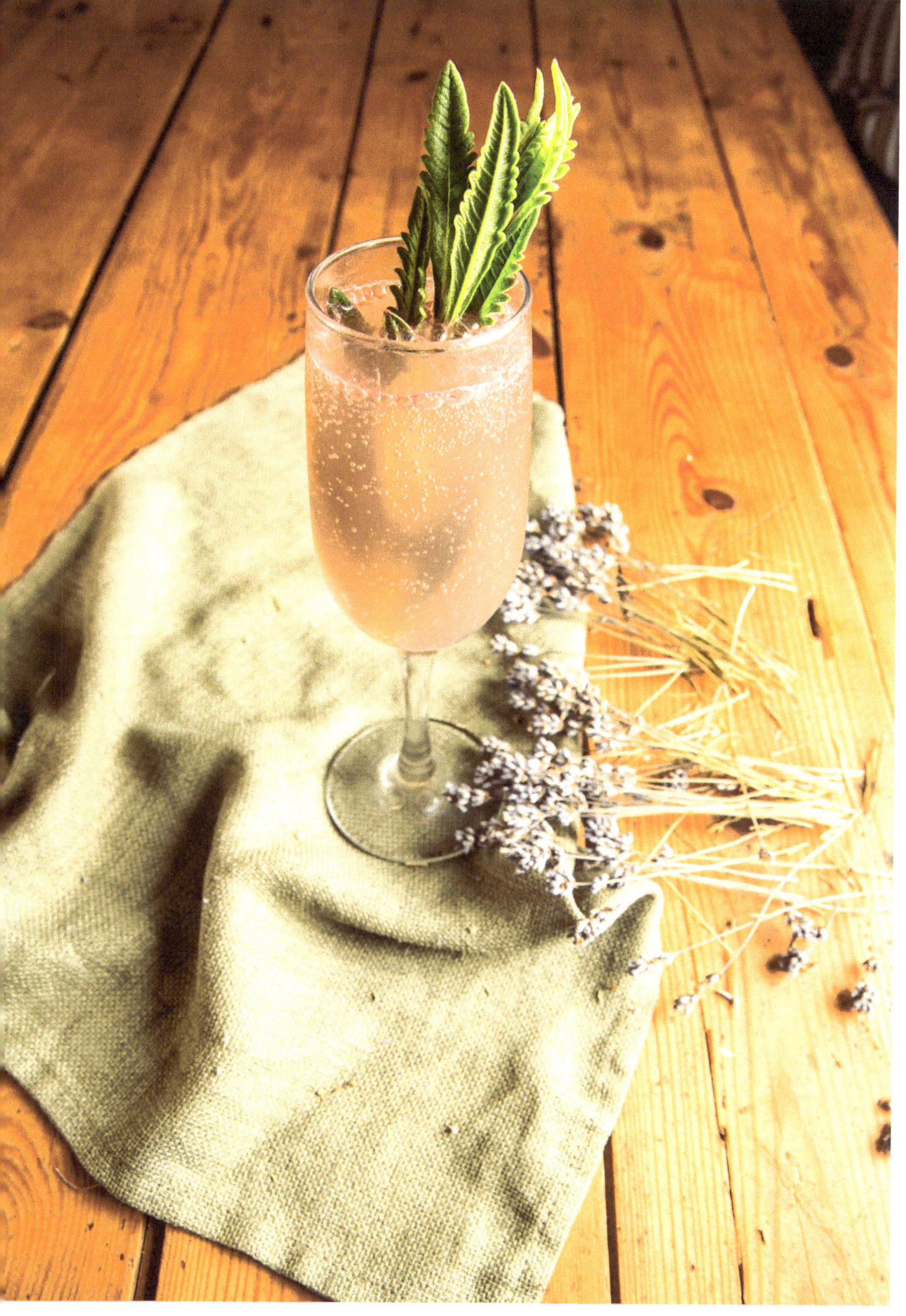

RECIPE BY BRIDESTOWE ESTATE LAVENDER

Chicken in French Mustard and Lavender Sauce

SERVES 4 FOR AN ENTREE OR LIGHT LUNCH

500 grams chicken pieces

2 rashers bacon

1 tablespoon plain flour

1 tablespoon olive oil

30 grams butter

4 onions

1 cup chicken stock

2 tablespoons dijon mustard

1 tablespoon Bridestowe Culinary Lavender

125ml cream

salt and freshly ground black pepper to taste

2 tablespoons chopped parsley

Toss the chicken pieces in the flour. Heat the butter and oil in a heavy casserole, add peeled and chopped onions and cook gently until soft. Remove from the pan. Add chicken and chopped bacon and brown. Add stock, salt, pepper, mustard and Bridestowe Culinary Lavender.

Return onions to the pan and bring slowly to the boil. Cover and simmer gently for 1 hour or until the chicken is tender. Remove the chicken and set aside on a warm serving plate then boil the sauce rapidly until it is slightly thickened. Adjust the seasoning, add the cream and parsley and pour the sauce over the chicken.

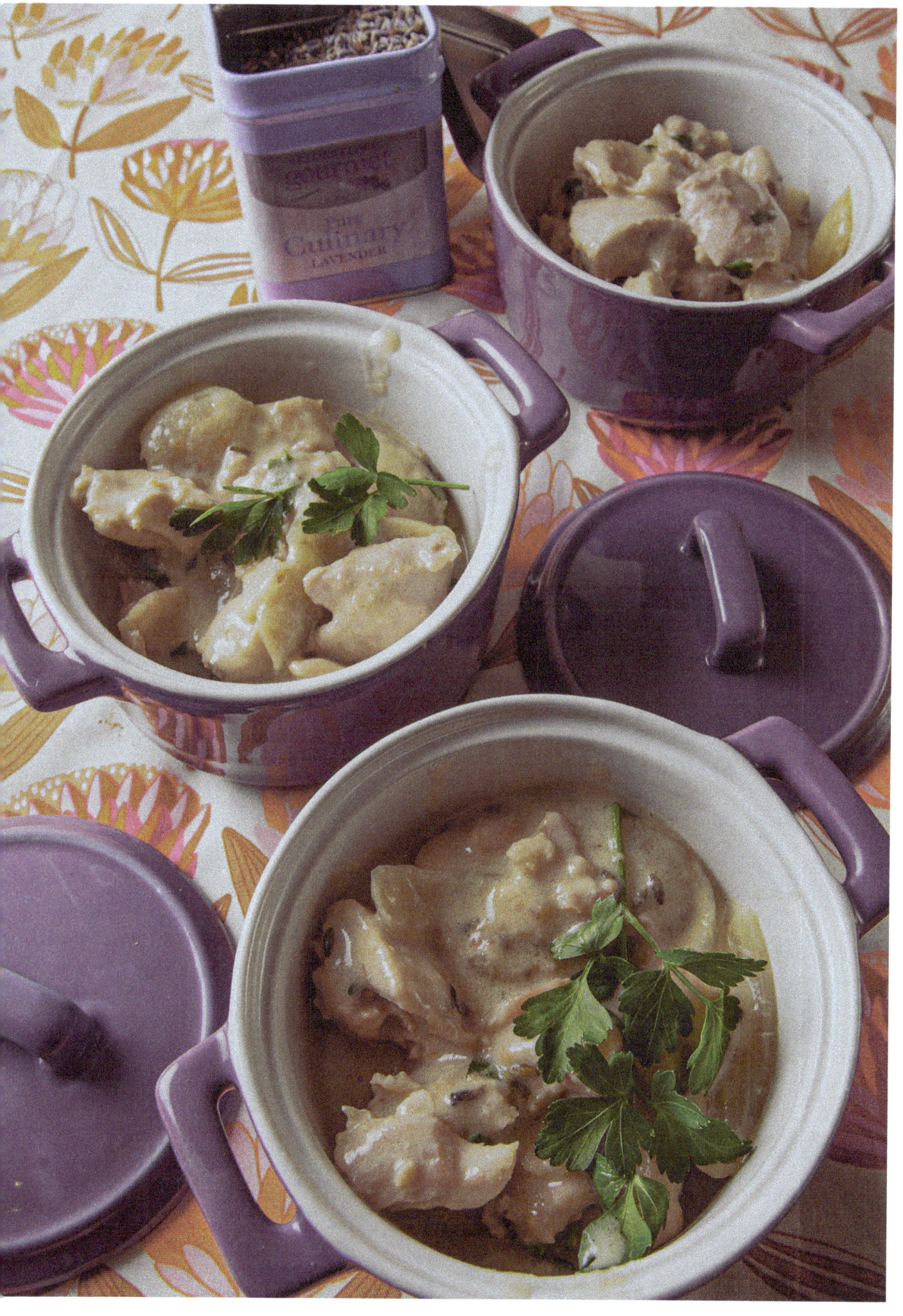

Slow Cooked Beef with Apple, Dijon, Lavender and Native Pepper

SERVES 4-6

800 grams oyster blade steak

¼ cup balsamic vinegar

1 cup white wine

1 cup vegetable or beef stock

3 small apples, peeled and chopped

1 large onion, finely chopped

2 cloves garlic, crushed

2 bay leaves

2 sprigs rosemary

2 sprigs thyme

1 tablespoon Dijon mustard

1 teaspoon dried culinary lavender

½ teaspoon ground native pepper (Tasmanian pepperberry)

1-2 tablespoons cornflour, mixed with a little cold water (optional, for thickening)

Brown the steak in a hot pan to seal, then place it in the slow cooker with the other ingredients. Cook on low for around six hours or until the meat is tender and falling apart. If you're serving it with wraps, salad or soft cheese, or want a thicker sauce, stir in the cornflour slowly and cook for another ten minutes with the lid off.

I thicken the sauce when serving it in wraps with honey mustard broccoli salad and soft goat's cheese, but I probably wouldn't bother if serving with mash, couscous or polenta to soak up all that beautiful aromatic sauce.

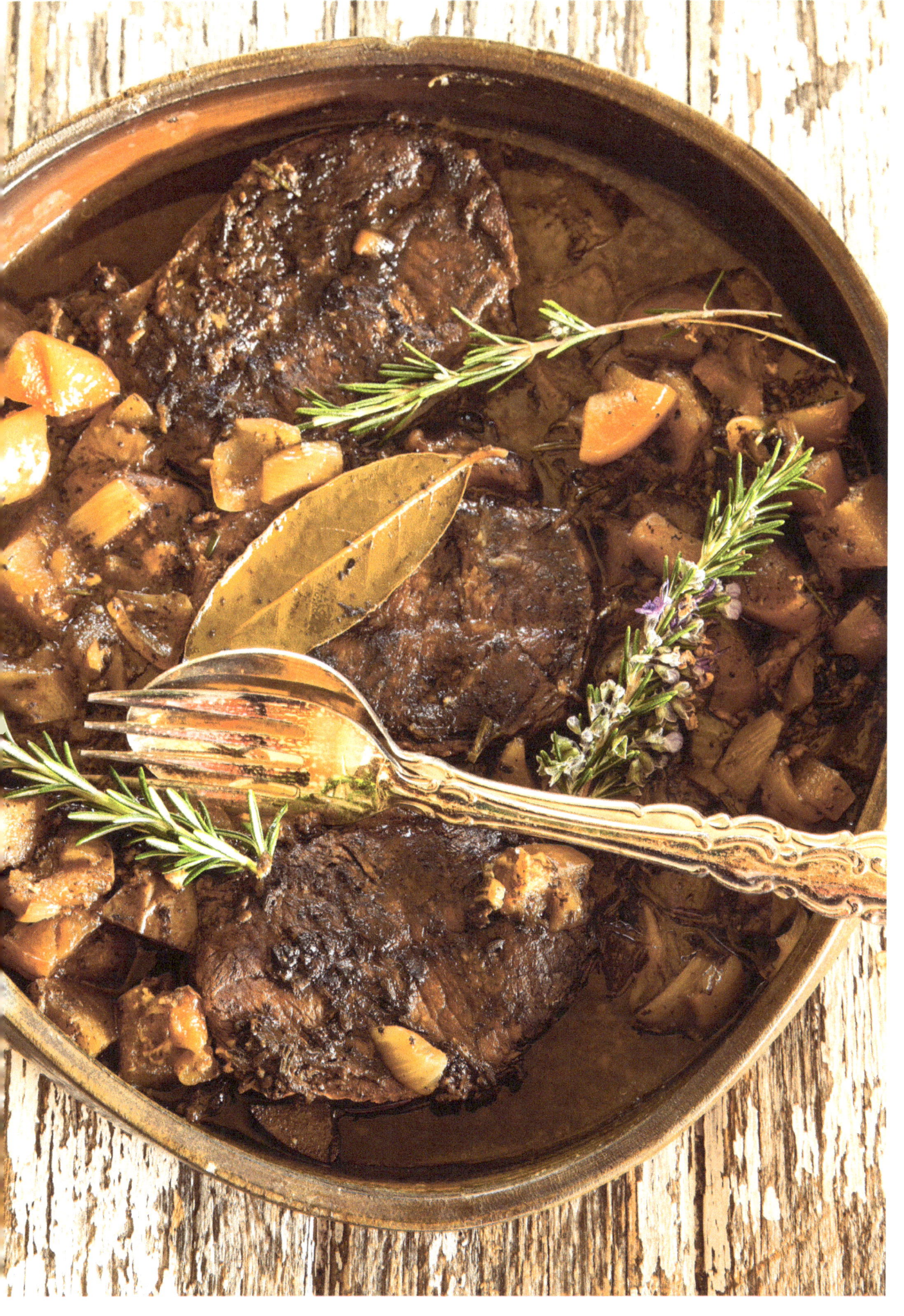

Smoked Fish Pate

MAKES ABOUT A CUP AND A HALF

100 grams cream cheese

1 tablespoon mayonaise

50ml cream

250 grams smoked fish

1 teaspoon dried culinary lavender

1 teaspoon dill

Put all ingredients in the blender and whiz together and serve, can be done the day before the event.

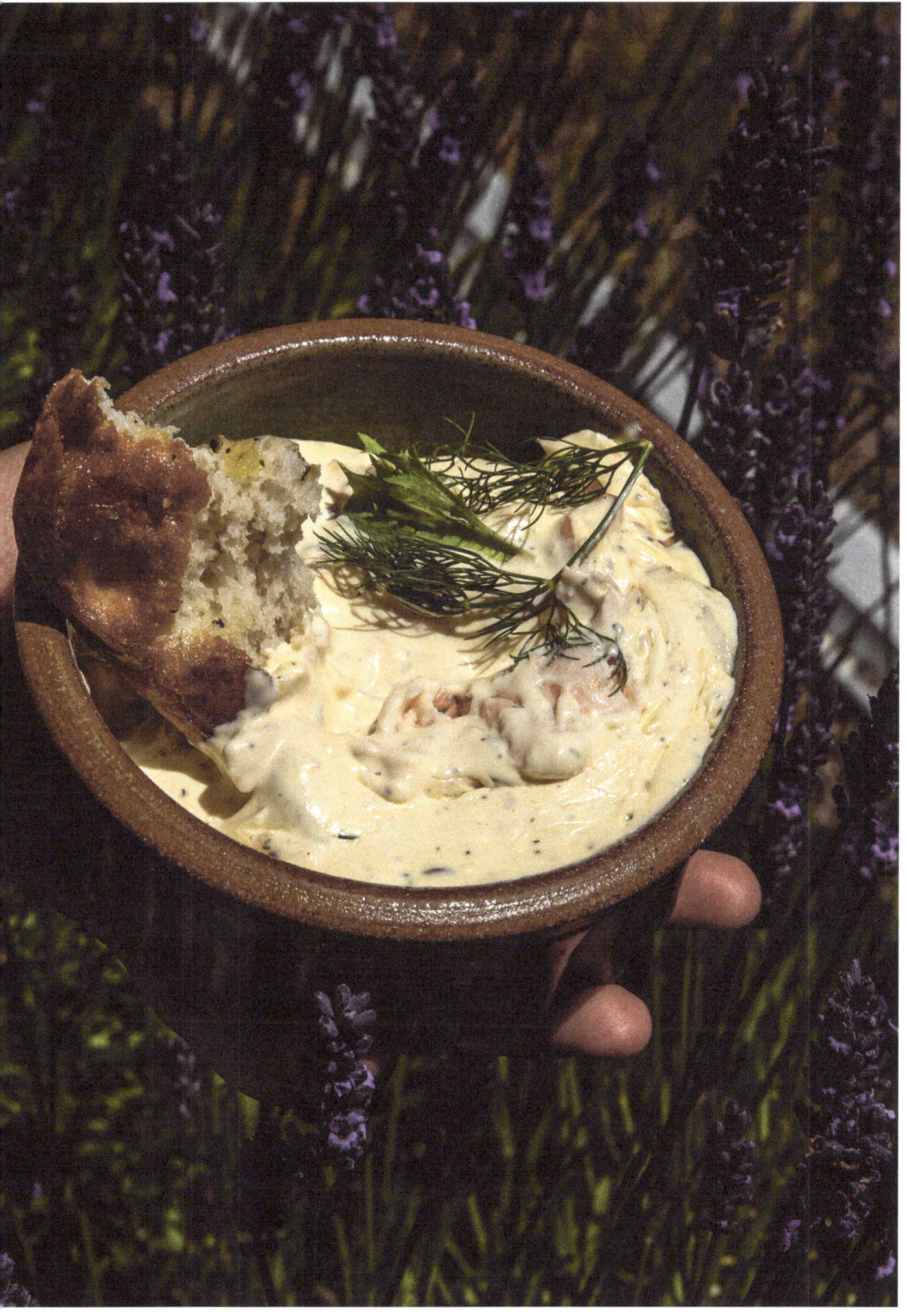

Slow Cooked Mediterranean Lamb Shoulder

MAKES A FEW FAMILY MEALS

Serve this delicious meat in a wrap with greek salad and yogurt.

approximately 2 kilo lamb shoulder

MARINADE

2 tablespoons extra virgin olive oil

6 cloves garlic

1 brown onion

1 sprig rosemary

4 sage leaves

2 teaspoons dry oregano

1 teaspoon dry basil

½ teaspoon pepper

1 teaspoon smoked paprika

1 teaspoon dry parsley

1 teaspoon dried culinary lavender and/or lavender leaf

Peel the garlic and onion and place in the thermocooker or food processor with all the marinade ingredients and blend until you make a smooth paste. Rub all over meat and pop in a lidded container and marinate in the fridge at least overnight.

Place the meat in the slow cooker and cook on high for around 5 hours or until you can pull all the meat apart with forks.

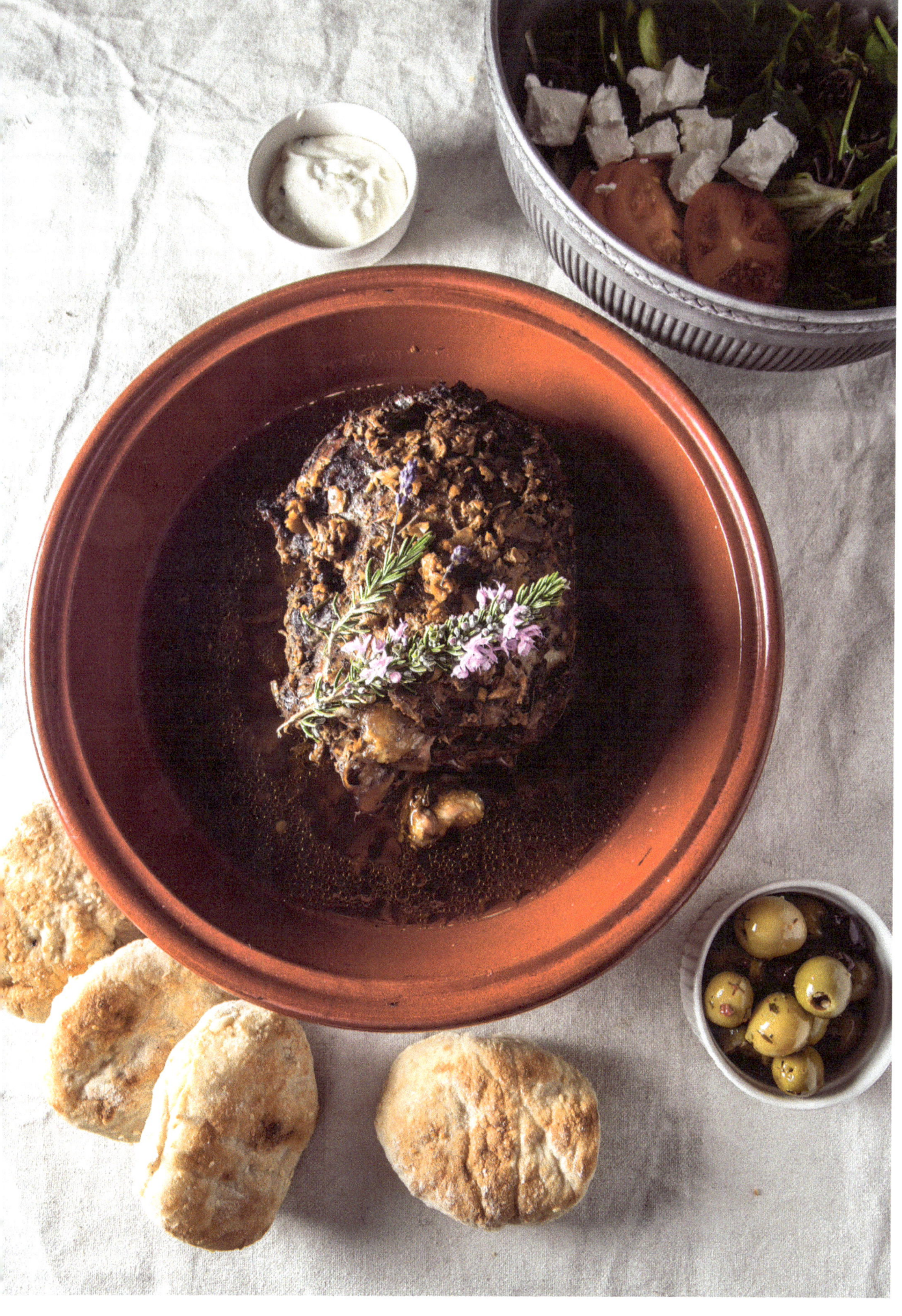

Pan-Fried Boarfish with Lavender and Blueberry Butter Sauce

SERVES 4

4 boneless boarfish fillets

sea salt

cracked black pepper

olive oil

butter, for frying

LAVENDER AND BLUEBERRY BUTTER SAUCE

150g unsalted butter, cold and diced

½ cup blueberries (fresh or thawed frozen)

1 teaspoon honey

½ teaspoon dried culinary lavender

1 small shallot, very finely diced

1 tablespoon red wine vinegar or verjuice

juice of half a lemon

pinch of sea salt

Season the fish fillets on both sides with sea salt and cracked black pepper and set them aside while you prepare the sauce.

In a small saucepan over low heat, soften the finely diced shallot in a little butter until translucent. Add the blueberries, lavender, and red wine vinegar or verjuice and let the mixture simmer gently until the blueberries start to break down and the liquid reduces slightly. Stir in the honey and lemon juice, then remove the pan from the heat. Whisk in the cold diced butter a few pieces at a time until the sauce becomes glossy and emulsified. Taste and add a pinch of salt or more lemon juice if needed. Keep warm but avoid reheating to prevent splitting.

Heat a wide pan over medium-high heat with a splash of olive oil and a knob of butter. Once hot and foaming, place the fish fillets skin-side down and press gently with a spatula to keep them flat. Cook for three to four minutes until the skin is crisp and golden, then flip and cook the other side for another one to two minutes until the fish is just cooked through.

Serve the fish skin-side up with the lavender and blueberry butter sauce spooned generously over the top. Garnish with extra blueberries or edible flowers if desired. This dish is lovely with soft polenta, creamy mashed potatoes, or steamed winter greens.

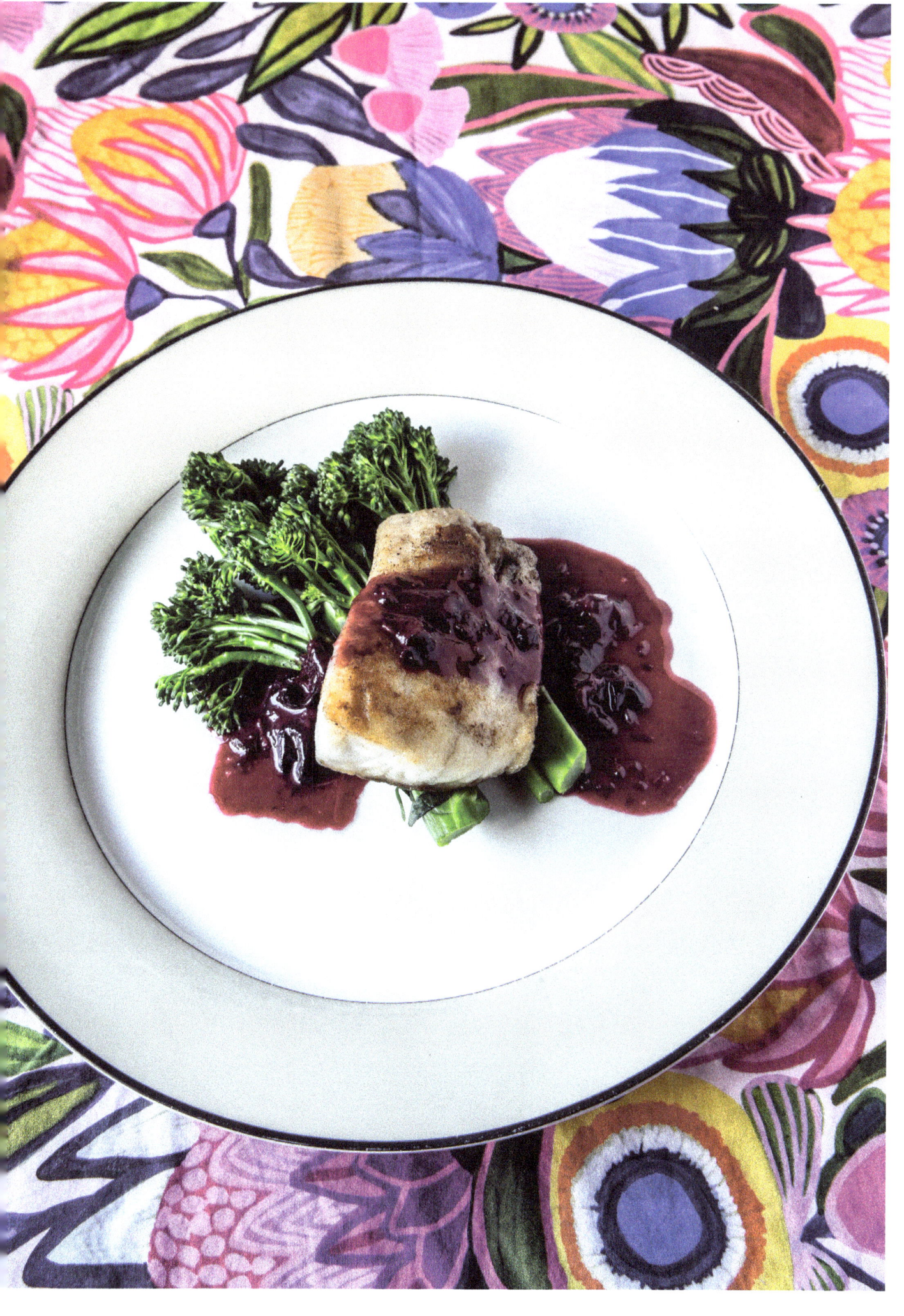

Grilled Octopus with Honey, Oregano, Lemon, Lavender and Garlic Marinade

SERVES 4-6

1 kilo octopus, cleaned

3 tablespoons honey

2 tablespoons fresh oregano leaves, finely chopped (or 1 tablespoon dried oregano)

juice and zest of 1 lemon

1 teaspoon dried culinary lavender

4 garlic cloves

4 tablespoons extra virgin olive oil

sea salt

cracked black pepper

Prepare the marinade by whisking together the honey, finely chopped oregano, lemon juice and zest, dried culinary lavender, crushed garlic, and extra virgin olive oil in a bowl. Season with sea salt and cracked black pepper to taste.

Cut the octopus into serving pieces and submerge them in the marinade. Cover and refrigerate for at least two hours, preferably overnight, so the garlic and herbs deeply infuse the flesh.

When ready to grill, preheat your grill or barbecue to medium-high. Remove the octopus pieces from the marinade, letting excess drip off, but keep a little marinade to brush during cooking. Grill the octopus for 3 to 4 minutes per side, allowing the honey to caramelise and the garlic to soften and infuse smoky flavour.

Serve the grilled octopus warm with a final drizzle of the reserved marinade and an extra squeeze of lemon. It's perfect alongside fresh salad greens, grilled vegetables, or simply with crusty bread.

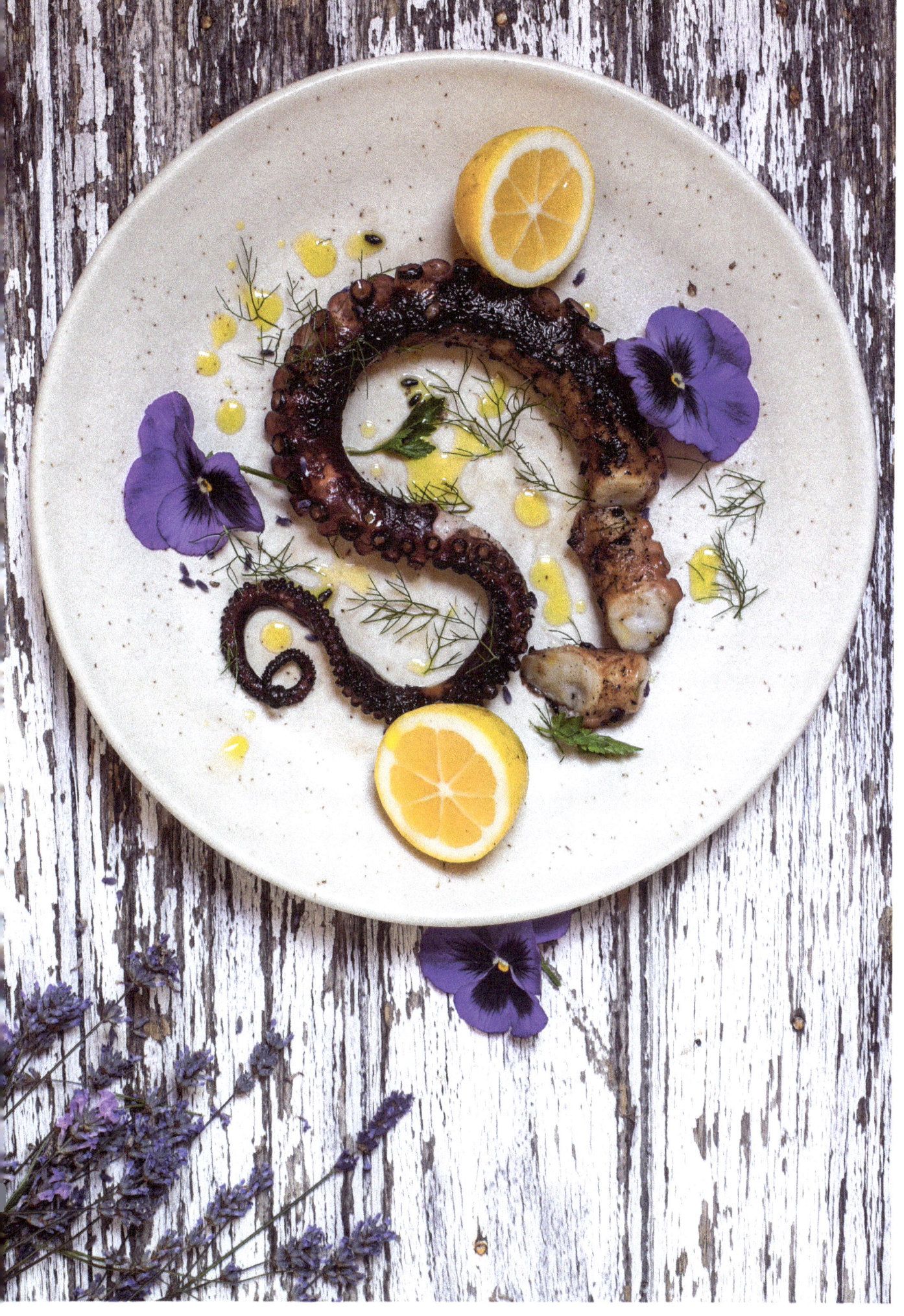

Lavender Custard Tart with Fruit

SERVES 6-8

FOR THE BASE

1 ½ cups flour

100 grams butter

2 tablespoons sugar

1 egg

FOR THE FILLING

320ml milk

1 teaspoon dried culinary lavender

a dash of vanilla essence

3 egg yolks

1 tablespoon sugar

1 tablespoon honey

2 tablespoons plain flour

3 tablespoons cornflour

500 grams strawberries or seasonal fruit

Preheat the oven to 180°C.

To make the pastry base, rub the butter into the flour and sugar with your fingertips until the mixture resembles fine crumbs. Add the egg and a tablespoon of cold water, then gently knead until it forms a smooth, firm dough. Wrap in baking paper or cling film and refrigerate for about an hour.

Grease and flour a 20cm tart tin with a removable base. Roll the chilled dough out on a cool, floured surface and gently line the base and sides of the tin. Patch any cracks with spare pastry and a little water if needed. Trim off the excess around the edges. Line the pastry with baking paper, fill with weights or rice, and bake blind for about 15 minutes or until golden. Remove from the oven and allow to cool. For the filling, gently heat the milk with the dried culinary lavender and a dash of vanilla. Once it reaches a gentle simmer, take it off the heat and let it infuse for 10 minutes. Strain out the lavender and return the milk to the pan.

In a large bowl, whisk together the egg yolks, sugar, honey, flour and cornflour until smooth. Slowly pour in the warm infused milk, whisking as you go. Return the mixture to the saucepan and cook over medium-low heat, stirring constantly until it thickens and begins to bubble. Let it cook for another minute to ensure the flour is cooked out, then remove from the heat.

Transfer the custard to a bowl, cover the surface with plastic wrap to stop a skin forming, and refrigerate until cold.

When ready to assemble, beat the chilled custard until smooth, spoon it into the tart shell, and top with strawberries or any seasonal fruit. Serve with a spoonful of cream, or just as it is.

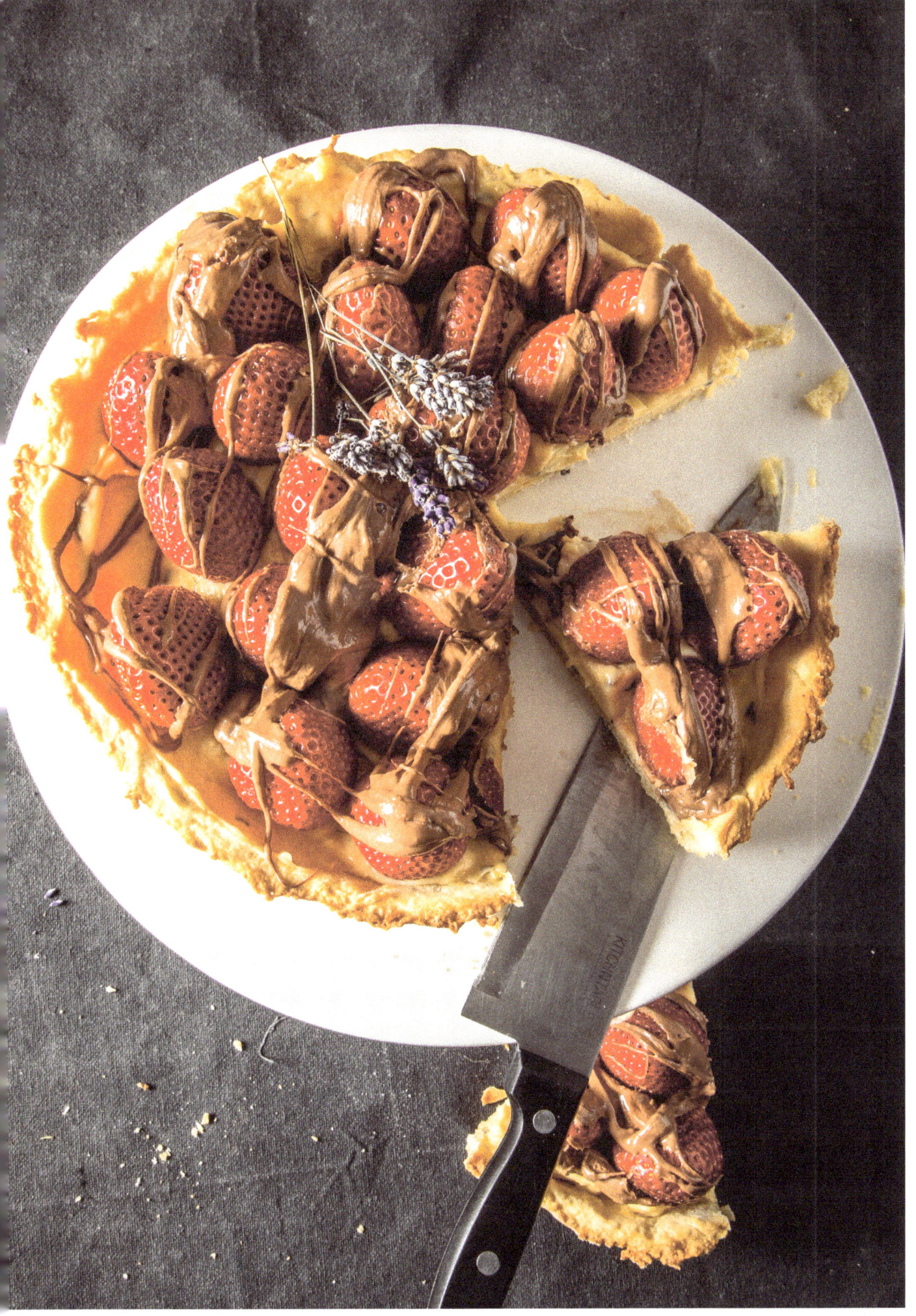

Honey and Lavender Dressed Apricot Chicken Summer Garden Salad

SERVES 2

FOR THE SALAD

2 small chicken breasts

1 tablespoon olive oil

6 fresh apricots (or 4 dried, soaked and sliced)

fresh green peas

1 small head of butter lettuce or mixed salad greens

1 small fennel bulb

½ avocado

40 grams creamy blue cheese

50 grams walnuts

fresh herbs like dill, parsely or tarragon

sea salt and cracked black pepper

FOR THE DRESSING

1 tablespoon honey

1 teaspoon dijon mustard

1 tablespoon lemon juice

2 tablespoons olive oil

¼–½ teaspoon dried culinary lavender

salt and pepper to taste

Steam the chicken breasts gently until just cooked—about 10-12 minutes—then allow to cool slightly before slicing.

To make the dressing, in a bowl, whisk the honey, lavender, Dijon mustard and lemon juice. Slowly add the lavender water and olive oil, whisking until emulsified. Season with salt and pepper to taste.

Arrange the lettuce and thinly sliced fennel on a serving platter. Add the sliced chicken, sliced apricots, avocado, peas, creamy blue cheese and walnuts. Scatter over the herbs. Drizzle with the lavender-infused dressing just before serving.

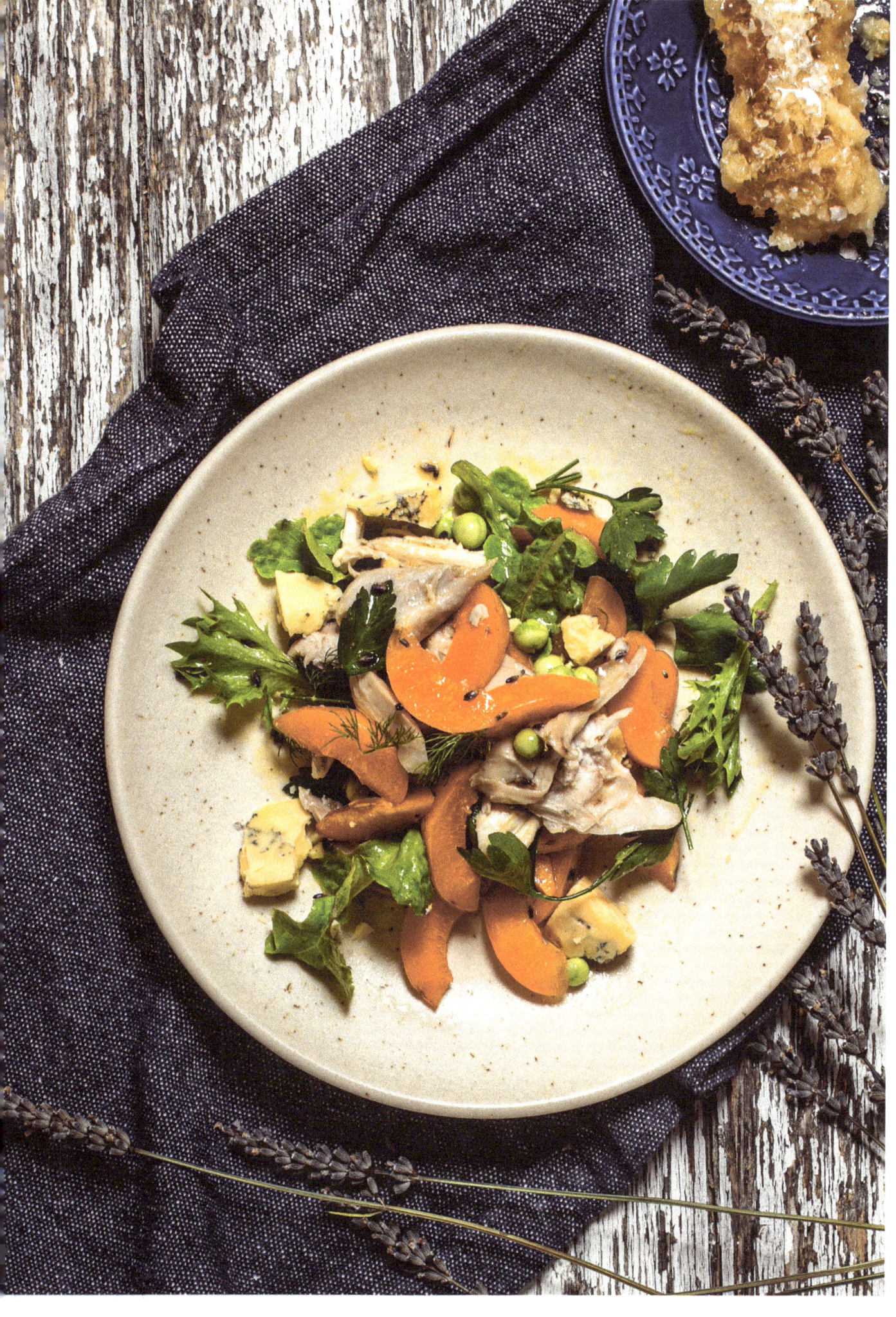

Apple, Cinnamon, Honey and Lavender Tea Cake

SERVES 6-8

100 grams butter

½ brown cup sugar

½ teaspoon vanilla essence

2 teaspoons dried culinary lavender

3 eggs

1 ½ cups self-raising flour

½ cup plain flour

200ml milk

1 teaspoon cinnamon

2 medium apples

2 tablesopoons honey

Beat the butter and sugar in a separate bowl until light and creamy and then beat in the eggs one at a time. Add the milk and then fold in the flour, vanilla, lavender and cinnamon. Grate the uncooked apples and fold through the mixture.

Pour the mixture into cupcake containers.

Bake in the oven for about 25 minutes or until golden brown and cooked through.

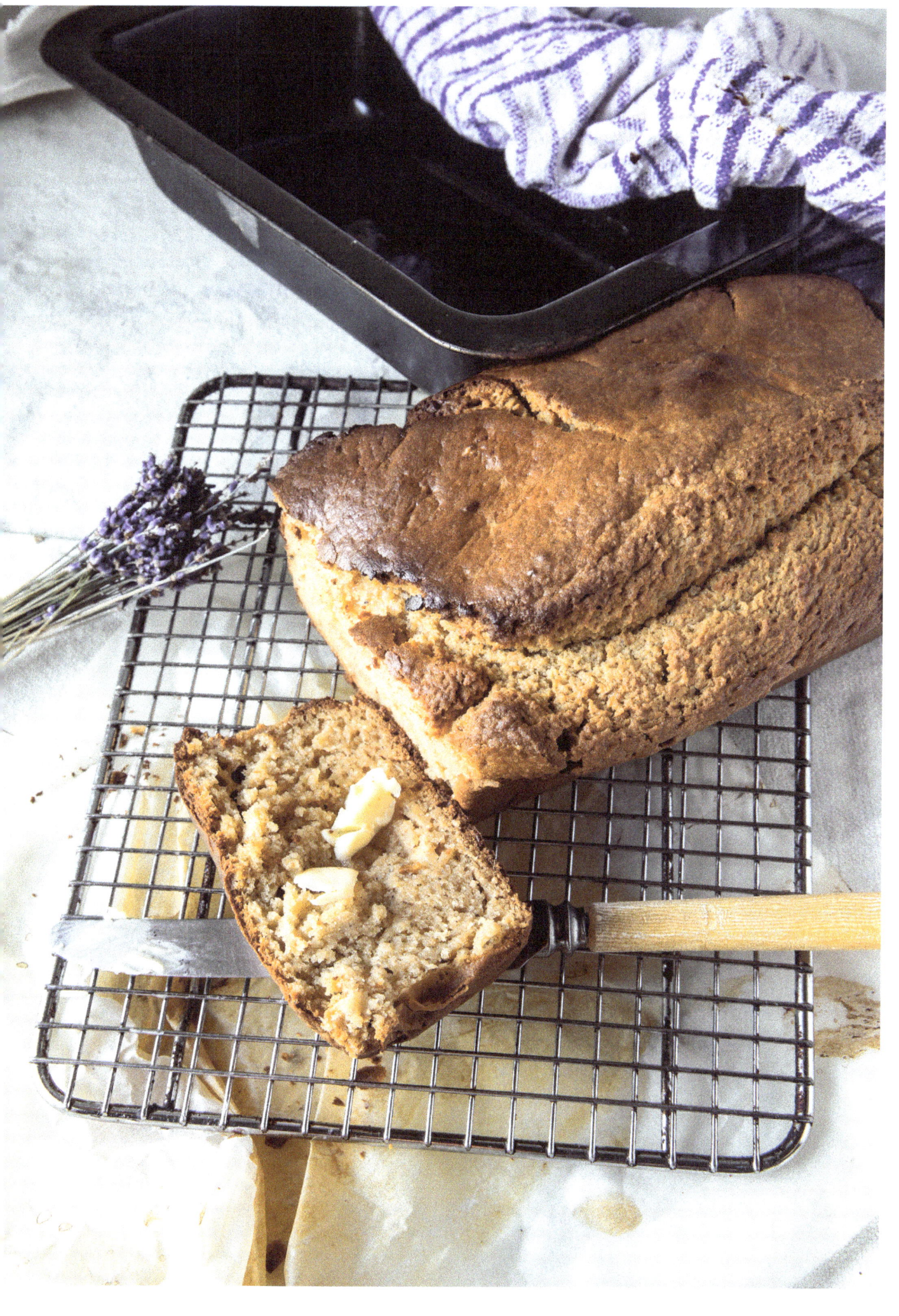

White Chocolate, Blueberry and Lavender Baked Cheesecake

SERVES 10

BASE

90 grams butter

120 grams flour

1 tablespoon sugar

1 ½ tablespoons water

FILLING

650 grams cream cheese

½ cup honey

½ cup sugar

3 eggs

½ cup plain flour

1 cup blueberries

1 teaspoon dried culinary lavender

1 ½ cups white chocolate

Line a 20cm spring form tin with baking paper and grease the sides.

Turn oven on to 175 °C.

In a food processor or in a bowl with your hands blend the flour, sugar and butter to produce fine crumbs. Add the water and knead into a firm dough. Press dough into the base of the tin.

Carefully melt the white chocolate in a bowl over a pot of simmering water.

Add the cream cheese to the food processor with the honey, eggs and sugar and whip until smooth. Add flour and whip through until smooth, whip through the melted white chocolate. Fold in the bluberries and lavender.

Pour onto the base and cook in a low oven until golden brown and cooked through.

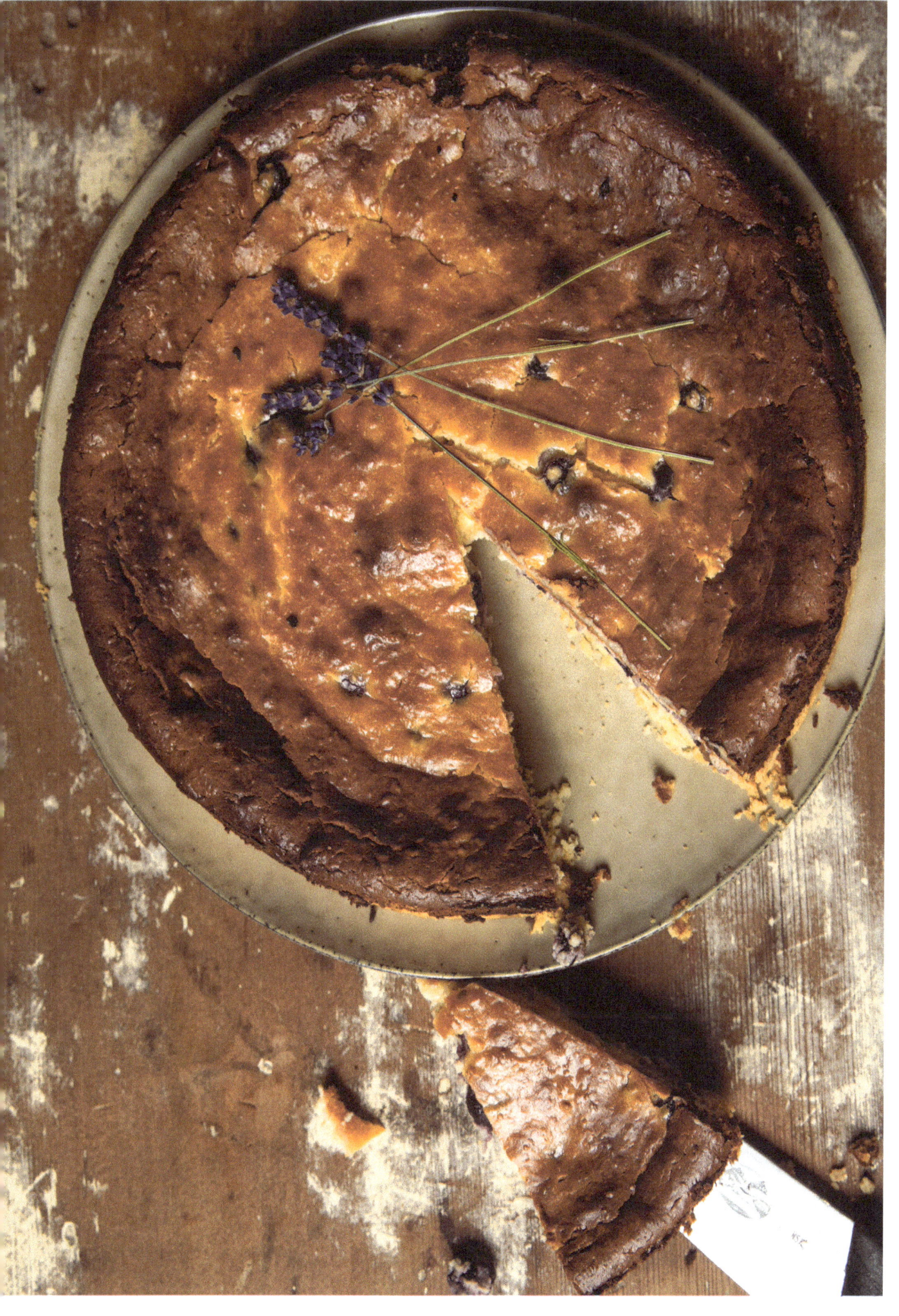

Foccacia with Herbs de Provence

MAKES ONE LARGE

500 grams strong white flour

1 teaspoon dried yeast

1 teaspoon sugar

1 teaspoon sea salt

350ml warm water

a generous pour of robust extra virgin olive oil

a fragrant blend of Herbs de Provence with a Tasmanian bush twist: wild oregano, saltbush, wild thyme, kunzea and a whisper of culinary lavender

In a large bowl, mix the flour, yeast, sugar and salt. Pour in the warm water and a splash of olive oil and mix to a shaggy dough. Turn out onto a lightly floured surface and knead by hand for 8–10 minutes until smooth and elastic. Place in a lightly oiled bowl, cover and let rise in a warm spot until doubled in size.

Transfer the dough to a well-oiled tray, stretch it gently to fit, and leave to rise again until puffed. Press your fingers deep into the dough to make dimples, drizzle generously with olive oil and sprinkle over the wild herb blend. Bake hot until golden and crisp on top, soft and steamy inside.

Best served still warm, with more oil for dipping.

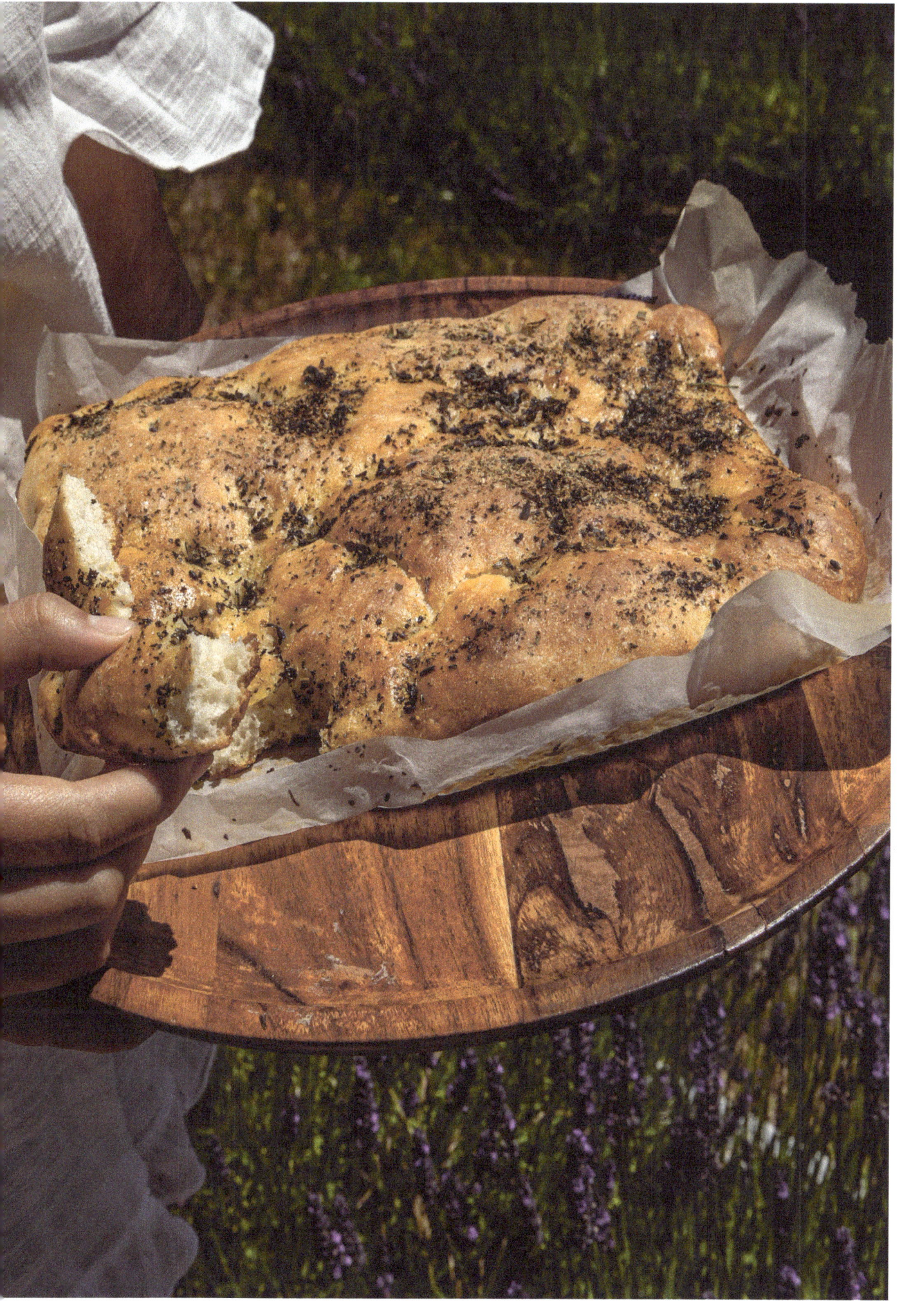

Granola with Lavender and Honey

SERVES 10

This stores well in an airtight container.

4 cups rolled oats
½ cup slivered almonds
¼ cup shredded or desiccated coconut
¼ cup seed sesame oil
1 teaspoon of grated lemon zest
1 teaspoon dried culinary lavender
½ cup extra virgin olive oil
1 cup chopped dried sultanas
4 tablespoons honey

Pre-heat the oven to 170°C. Mix together the oats, nuts, desiccated coconut, seeds, lavender and lemon zest. Warm the oil, honey and syrup in a saucepan on the stove. Pour the syrup mixture into the oat mixture and mix well.

Divide the mixture on to 2 large baking dishes and bake, stirring every 5 minutes for 20 minutes until golden.

Cool then stir through the dried fruit.

Serve with milk or yogurt for breakfast

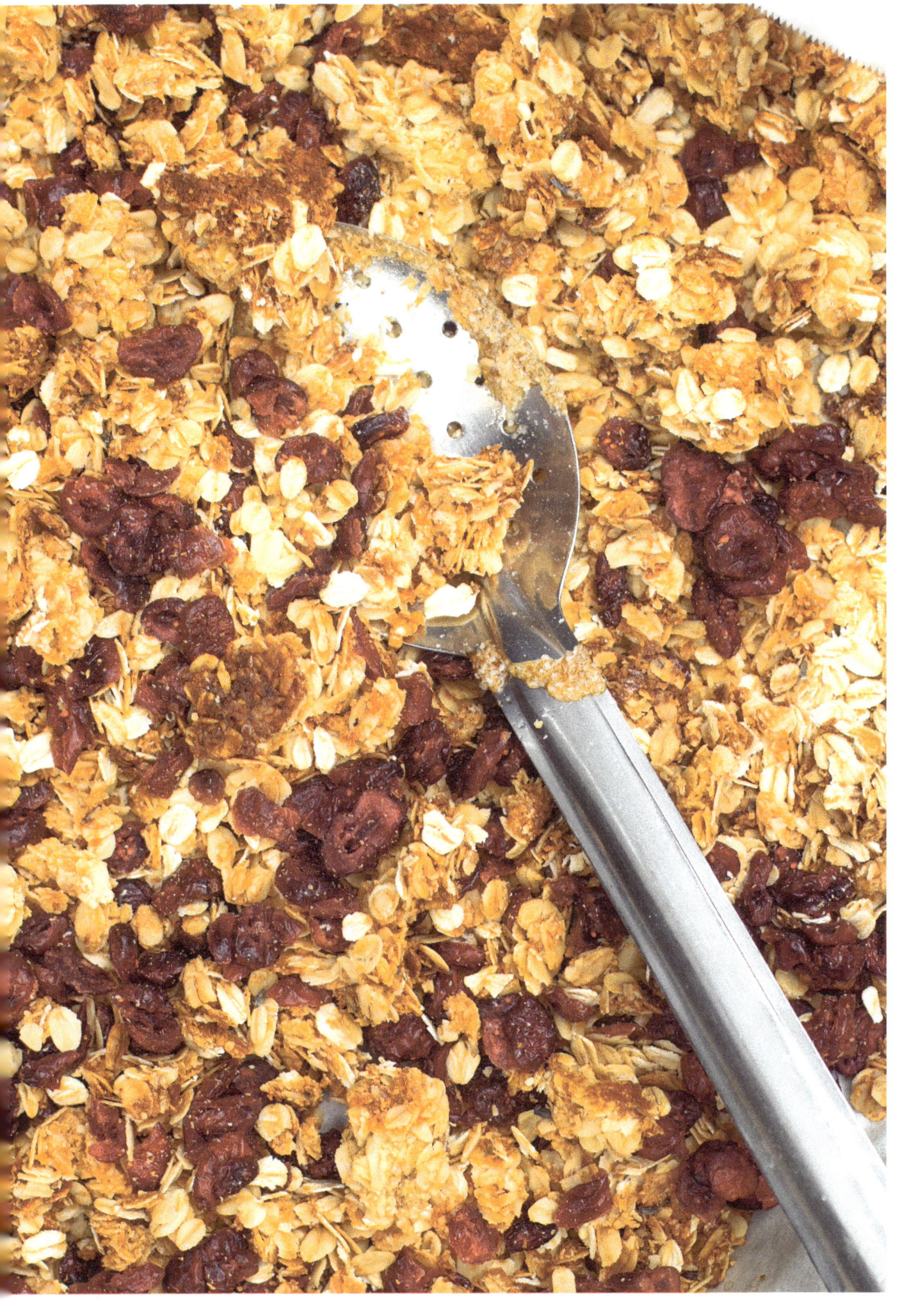

Apple and Lavender Crumble

SERVES 6

Substitute the butter for extra virgin olive oil. A lemon agrumato oil adds a refreshing flavour to the crumble. Replace the stewed apples with any presevred fruits and mix with berries. And use any preserved, tinned or fresh fruits that you like.

6 large apples

1 tablespoon sugar

120 grams self-raising flour

100 grams brown sugar

80 grams butter

60 grams rolled oats

½ teaspoon dried culinary lavender

Turn the oven on to 180°C. Peel and remove the core from the apples and cut them into a 1cm dice.

Place the diced apples into a heavy based saucepan with a lid and over a low heat stew for about 10 minutes until soft. Pour the stewed apple into a casserole dish.

To make the crumble, first rub the butter and flour together to make the base and then add the oats, brown sugar and lavender. Mix well and then put on top of the apple. Bake the crumble for about 20 minutes until golden brown.

Serve with ice- cream or cream.

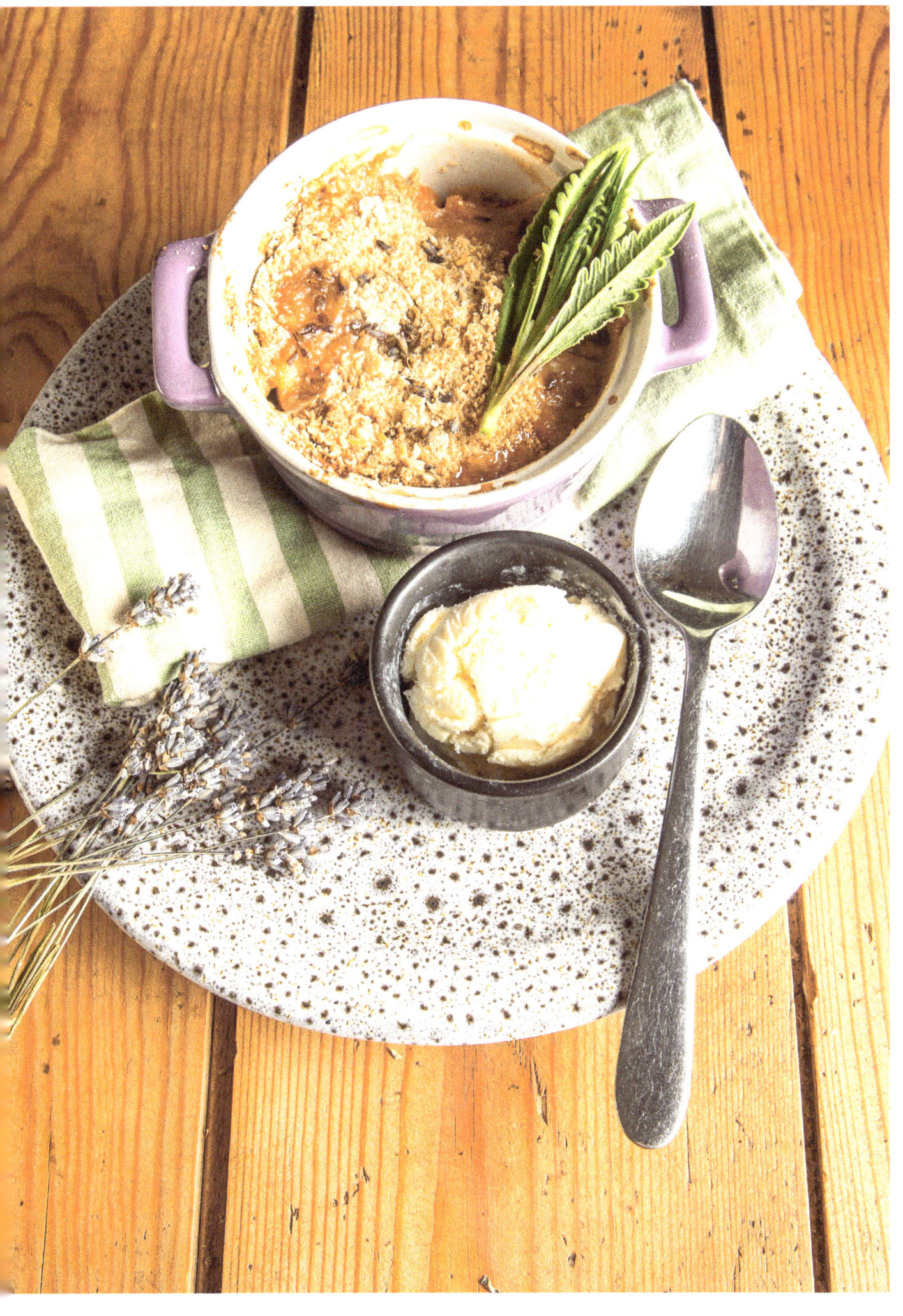

Steamed Parrot Fish, Dijon, Lemon, Mandarin and Lavender

SERVES 2

A big fish or 2 in the centre of the table is a great way to feed a group.

one large parrot fish

2 tablespoons robust and fresh extra virgin olive oil

3 mandarins

2 tablespoons dijon mustard

1 teaspoon dried culinary lavender

2 tablespoons lemon juice

sea salt

pepper

Steam the fish in a fish poacher. If you do not have a fish poacher simply use a baking tray half filled with water, with a cake rack to fit the fish on and foil over the top or a tight fitting lid if you have one. This set up on the stove top will work well. The fish is going to take at least 20 minutes to steam gently. But it all depends on the size. The fish is cooked when the flesh can easliy be scrapped from the frame. Alternatively the fish can be cooked in foil lined with baking paper and wrapped up tightly, to steam the fish in the oven.

To make the sauce, peel the mandarins. Whisk all the other sauce ingredients together and add the peeled mandarin and season well with salt and pepper. Pour dressing over the cooked fish.

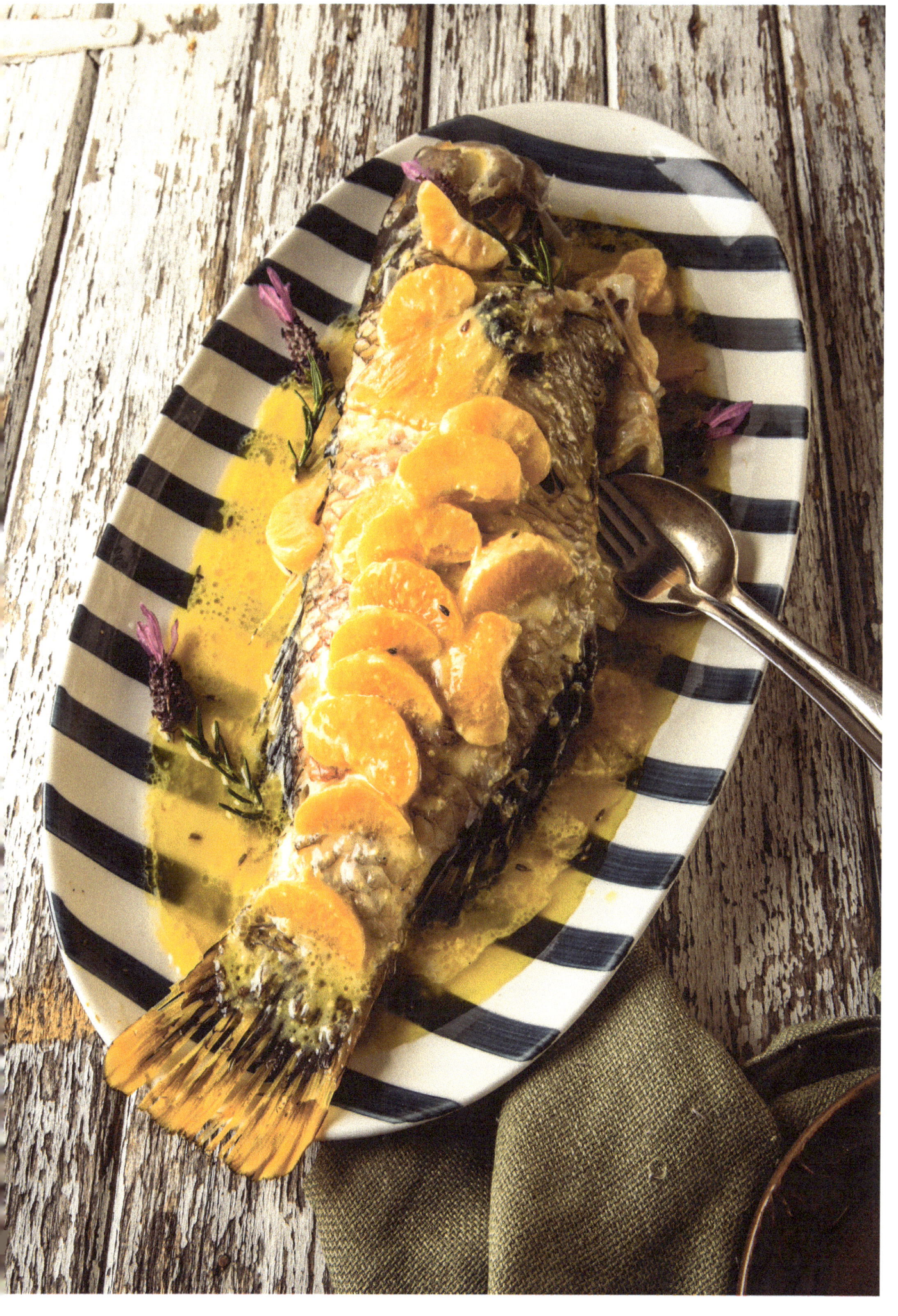

Burnt Butter, Rosemary, Lavender and Honey Cake

MAKES A DOUBLE LAYER CAKE THAT SERVES ABOUT 16

FOR THE CAKE

250 grams unsalted butter

1 tablespoon finely chopped fresh rosemary

1 tablespoon honey

1 teaspoon dried culinary lavender

1 cup caster sugar

4 eggs

1 teaspoon vanilla extract

2¼ cups self-raising flour

½ cup milk

FOR THE BUTTERCREAM

200 grams unsalted butter

3 cups icing sugar

½ teaspoon dried culinary lavender

½ teaspoon vanilla paste or extract

Heat 100 grams of butter gently in a small saucepan until it froths and goes golden and nutty, stirring often.. Add the rosemary and let it sizzle for a moment. Off the heat, stir in the honey and lavender and let it cool until soft but not firm.

Cream the cooled burnt butter mixture and the remaining butter with the sugar until light. Beat in the eggs one at a time, followed by vanilla. Fold in the flour alternately with the milk.

Bake in 2 small lined cake tin at 170°C until golden and just springing back—about 35-45 minutes depending on your pan. Cool completely before icing.

For the buttercream, beat the butter until creamy and add icing sugar, vanilla and lavender. Whip until pale, fluffy.

Ice generously, decorate simply—maybe with a few dried culinary lavender buds, rosemary sprigs, or a little extra drizzle of honey. This one keeps beautifully and tastes even better the next day.

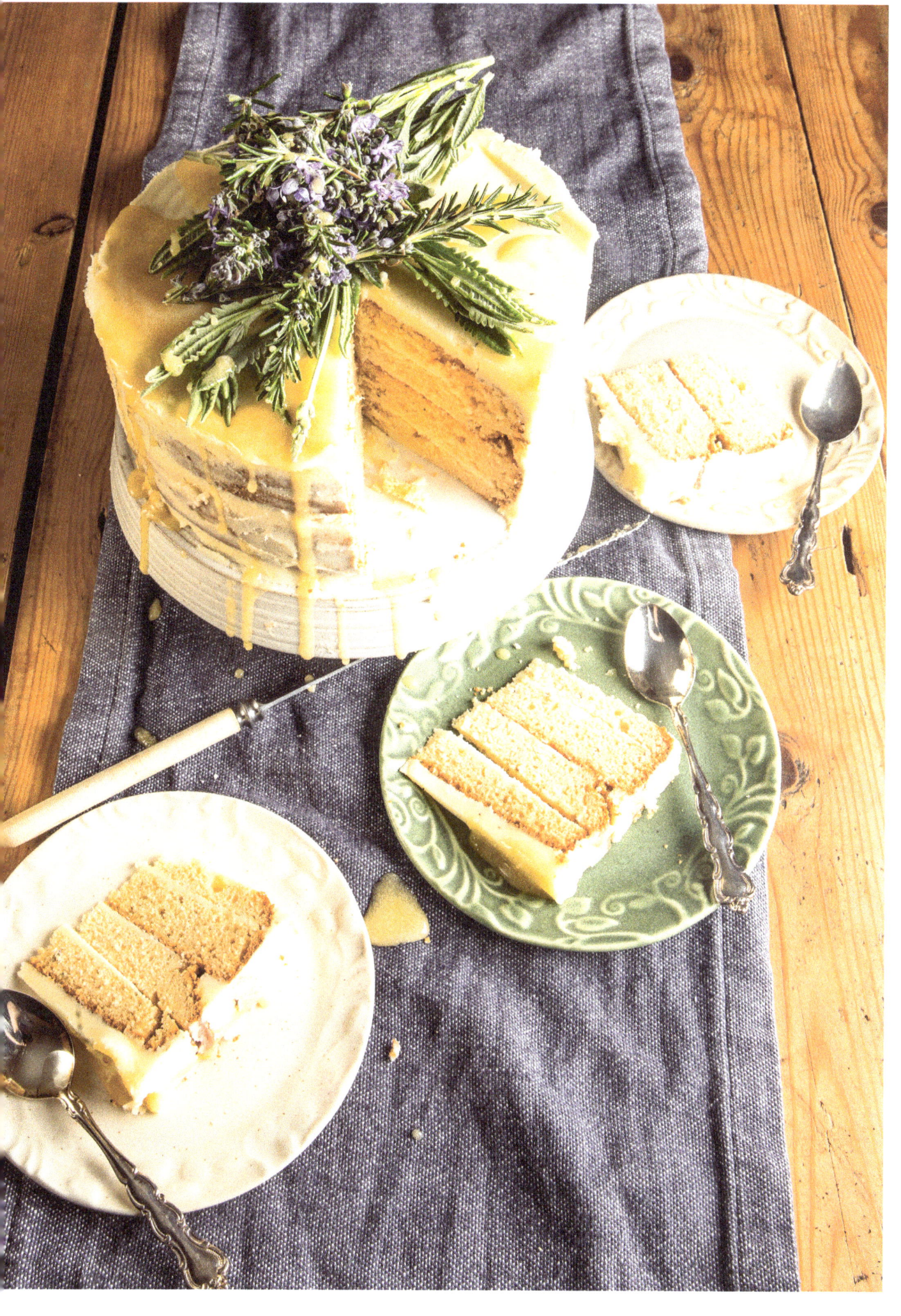

Blackberry Lavender Syrup

MAKES ABOUT HALF A LITRE

With some ice cream and lemonade this syrup makes a delicious and fun spider.

1½ cups fresh or frozen blackberries

1 cup water

¾ cup sugar (or ½ cup honey for a softer flavour)

1 teaspoon dried culinary lavender

1 teaspoon lemon juice

Combine blackberries, water, sugar (or honey), and lavender in a small saucepan. Bring to a simmer over medium heat, stirring gently. Let it bubble away for 10–15 minutes, crushing the berries slightly with a spoon as they soften.

Take off the heat, stir in the lemon juice, and let it soak for 10 more minutes. Strain through a fine sieve or muslin—pressing to extract all the juice. Bottle and chill.

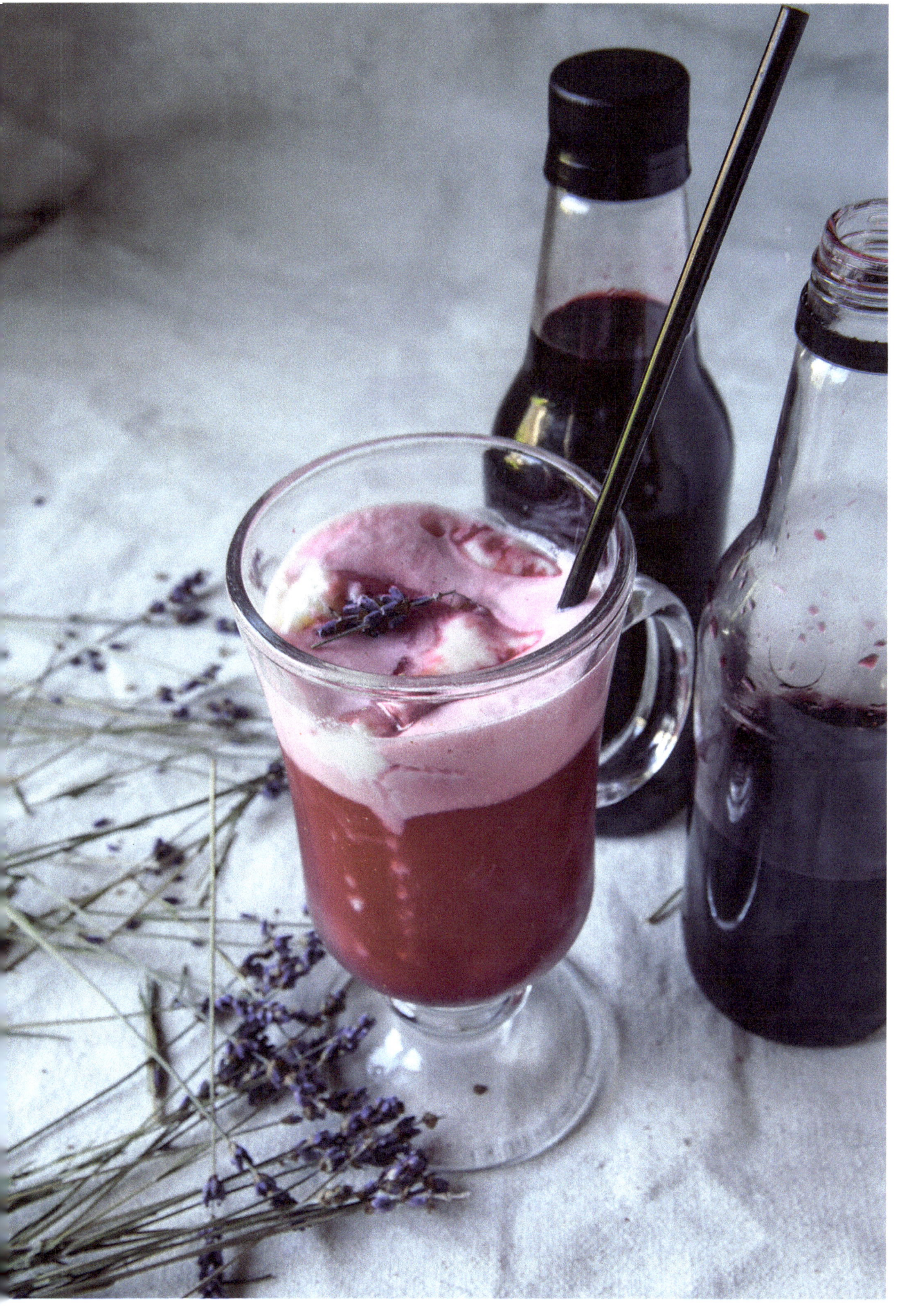

Creme Brulee with Lavender and Raspberry

SERVES SIX ONE LARGE OR 6 SMALL

Pretty much any stewed fruit or fresh berry can be used in this brulee recipe. You will need a kitchen blow torch to finish the brulee off and get the good caramelised sugar top. Do not be shy with your sprinkle of sugar on top, a nice thick toffee on top is always good and take your time with the blow torch, I find waving it over in circles works well so there are no burnt bits. The brulee can be served hot or cold.

200 grams raspberry

½ teaspoon dried culinary lavender

1 cup cream

1 cup milk

1/3 cup sugar

vanilla bean split

3 eggs

sugar to caramelise on top

Preheat the oven to 150°C

Put the milk and cream in a heavy based pot, split the vanilla bean and scrape into the milk and cream and bring to a gentle simmer, add the lavender. Remove from heat.

Beat the eggs and the sugar in a large bowl until creamy and beat in the hot milk and cream. Beat well.

Place the raspberries at the base of the brulee mould you want to use, 6 small or one large, and pour the cream and milk mix on top.

Put the moulds into a water bath in a roasting tray the water should come at least of the way up the sides of the moulds, bake for about 30 minutes at 150°C or until set and cooked.

Cool. Sprinkle with sugar and caramelise the sugar with a blow torch and serve with icecream or cream.

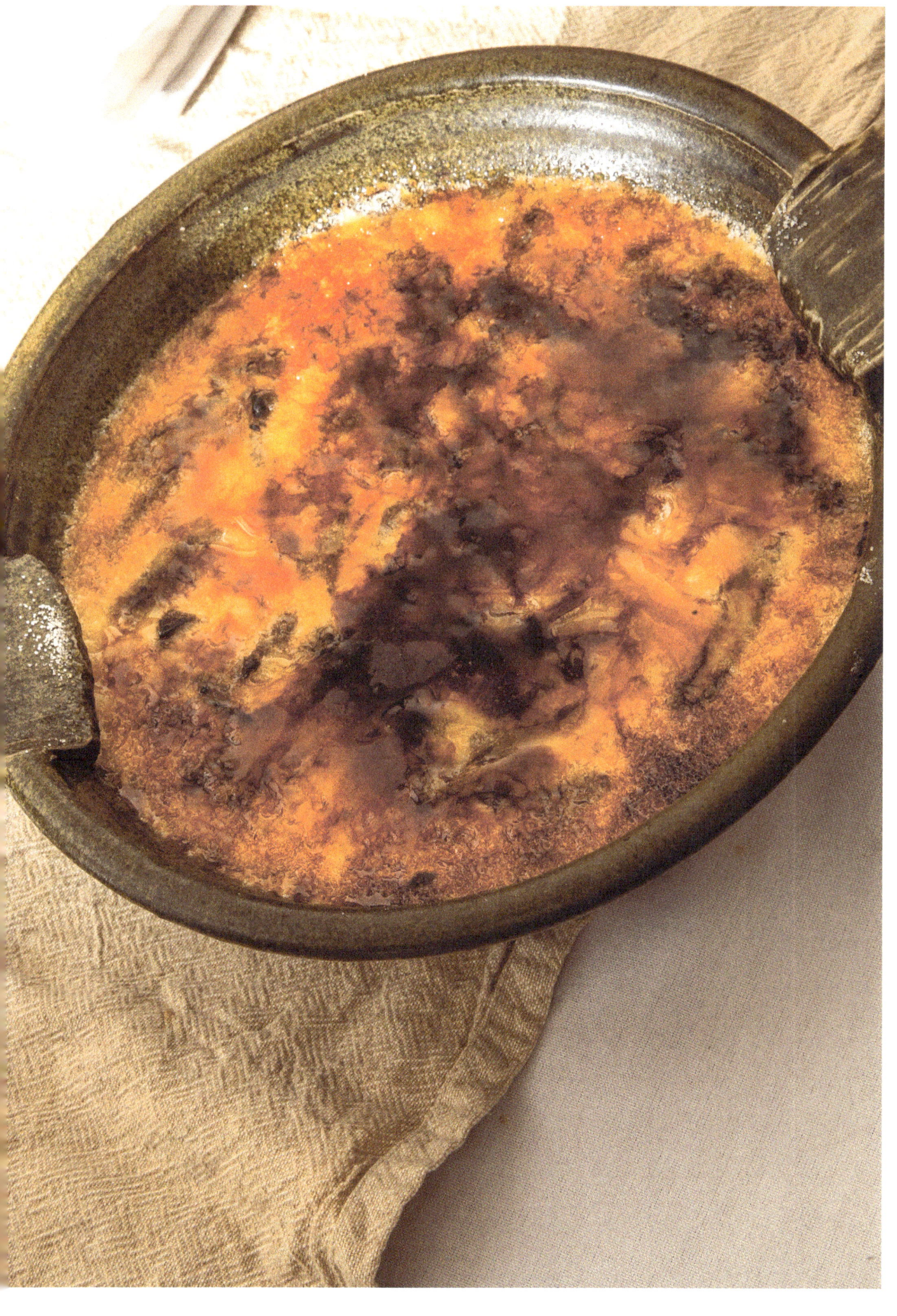

Pork Loin with Honey, Mustard and Lavender Sauce

SERVES 4

A beautiftul rich sauce for pork steak that could also be served with roatsed or slow cooked pork. This sauce can also be served with chicken, quail or fish.

4 pork loin steaks

½ onion

1 clove garlic

1 teaspoon butter

2 cups cream

1 tablespoon honey

1 teaspoon mustard

½ teaspoon dried culinary lavender

Cook the pork loin steaks in a medium hot pan or on the BBQ, with a drizzle of extra virgin olive oil until just cooked through and rest.

Peel and dice onion, crush garlic and saute in a heavy based pan and all the other ingredients and season with salt and pepper. Simmer over a low heat until the sauce has reduced and thickened. Serve with some roast or mashed vegtables or salad.

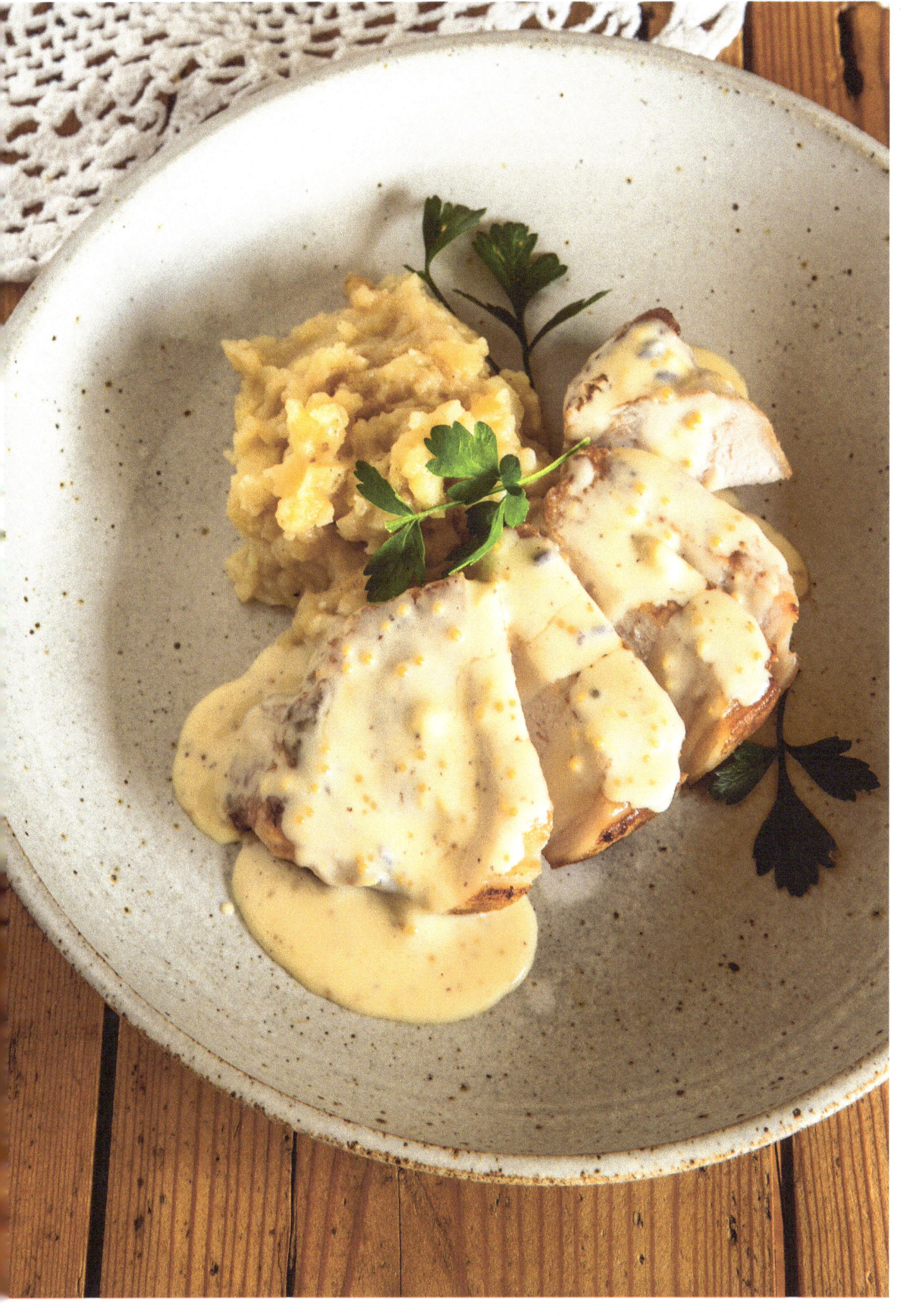

Mackeral Baked with Lemon, Olive Oil, Lavender and Bush Herbs

SERVES 2

2 whole mackerel, cleaned and scaled or filleted

1 lemon, sliced thinly

juice of ½ lemon

splash extra virgin olive oil

½ teaspoon dried culinary lavender

½ teaspoon native pepperberry, crushed

½ teaspoon dried saltbush

½ teaspoon wild thyme or native thyme

sea salt

Preheat the oven to 200°C. Score the mackerel on both sides and lay them in a baking dish. Drizzle generously with olive oil and lemon juice, season with sea salt.

Rub the lavender, pepperberry, saltbush, and wild thyme into the fish and scatter more over the top. Tuck lemon slices into the cavities and in the slits of the fish.

Bake uncovered for 20-25 minutes, until the skin blisters slightly and the flesh is cooked through.

Serve warm, drizzled with the pan juices—maybe with steamed potatoes, wilted greens or some warm crusty bread to mop it all up.

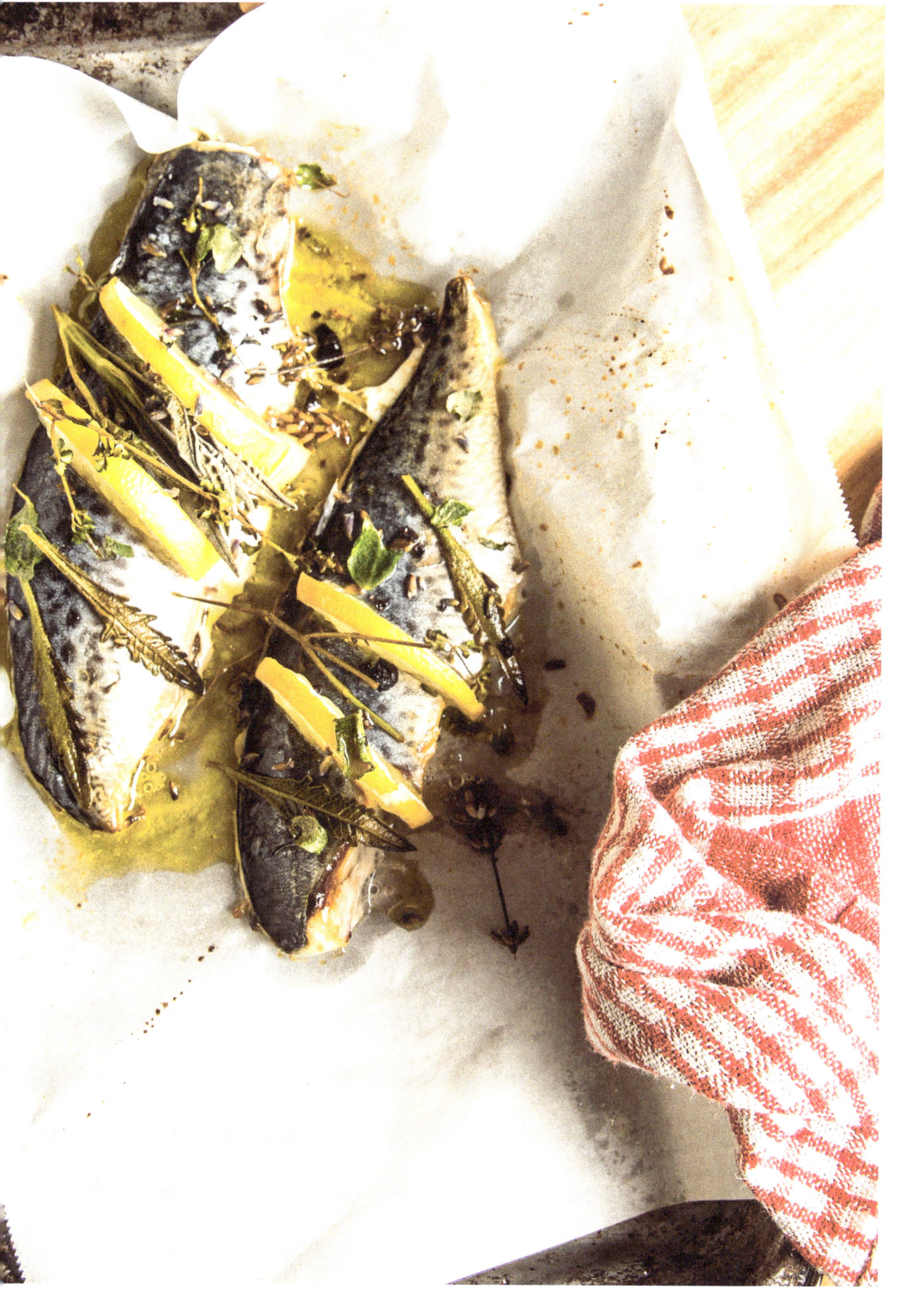

Chicken with Quince and Lavender

SERVES 4

6 chicken thighs

2 brown onions

2 quinces- preserved or poached

1 teaspoon dried culinary lavender

1 tablespoon honey

½ teaspoon ground native pepperberry or black pepper

splash extra virgin olive oil

spinch sea salt

splash of white wine or verjuice

a little water or chicken stock

Season the chicken thighs with salt and pepper. Brown them in olive oil, skin-side down first, until golden. Set aside.

In the same pan, lower the heat and add the onions. Cook slowly until soft and caramelised. Add the quince slices and let them take on some colour. Stir in the lavender, honey, pepperberry and a splash of wine or verjuice. Let it bubble up and reduce slightly.

Return the chicken to the pan, nestling it in among the onions and quince. Add a little water or stock, cover tightly with a lid or foil, and slow cook at 160°C for about 1½ hours, or until the chicken is tender and the quince is soft and fragrant.

Uncover for the last 15–20 minutes to allow the juices to thicken slightly.

Serve with creamy mash, soft polenta or warm flatbread to soak up the syrupy pan juices. The lavender should be subtle—more of a warmth in the background than a strong note.

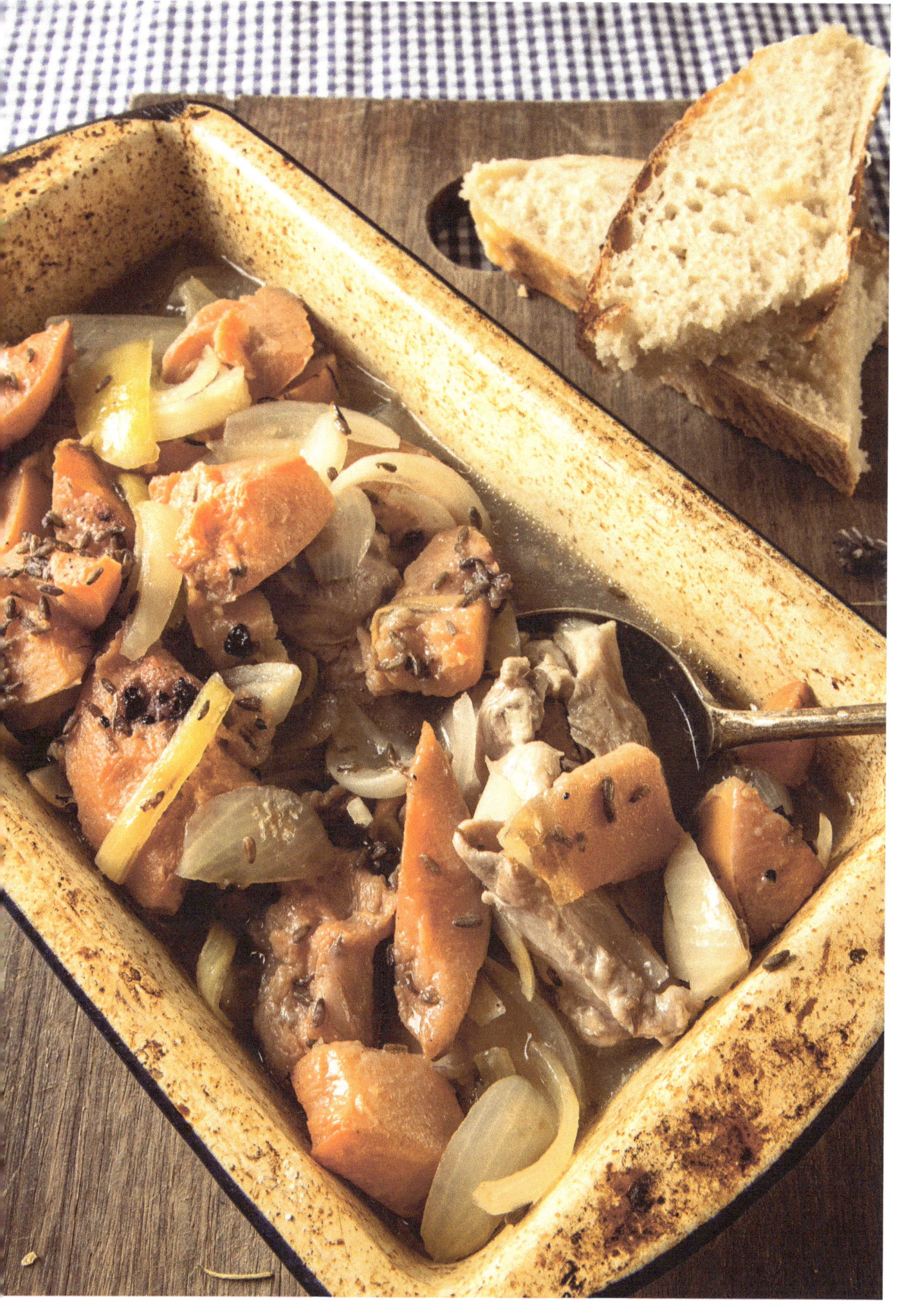

Chocolate Ricotta and Lavender Pie

SERVES 8

PASTRY

2 cups self-raising flour

¼ cup caster sugar

125 grams butter

½ cup milk

FILLING

500 grams ricotta

3 eggs

¾ cup sugar

80 grams dates

120 grams dark chocolate

zest of 1 lemon

1 teaspoon cinnamon

1½ teaspoons dried culinary lavender

Start by making the pastry. In a large bowl, combine the self-raising flour and caster sugar. Cut the butter into small cubes and rub it into the flour with your fingertips until it resembles coarse breadcrumbs. Pour in the milk gradually, stirring gently with a butter knife or your hands until the dough just comes together. Turn it out onto a lightly floured surface and knead briefly until smooth. Wrap and chill the dough for about 30 minutes while you prepare the filling.

For the filling, place the ricotta in a mixing bowl and beat in the eggs and sugar until smooth and light. Roughly chop the dates and dark chocolate and fold them through the mixture. Add the finely grated lemon zest, cinnamon, and crushed lavender, mixing well to combine all the flavours.

Preheat your oven to 180°C (fan-forced 160°C). Roll out the chilled pastry on a floured surface and line a tart tin (around 24cm) with the dough, pressing it gently into the edges and trimming the excess. Spoon the ricotta filling into the pastry case and smooth the top.

Bake for about 35–40 minutes, or until the filling is just set and lightly golden on top. Allow the tart to cool slightly before serving. It's beautiful warm or cold, with a dollop of cream or yoghurt, or simply with a pot of tea.

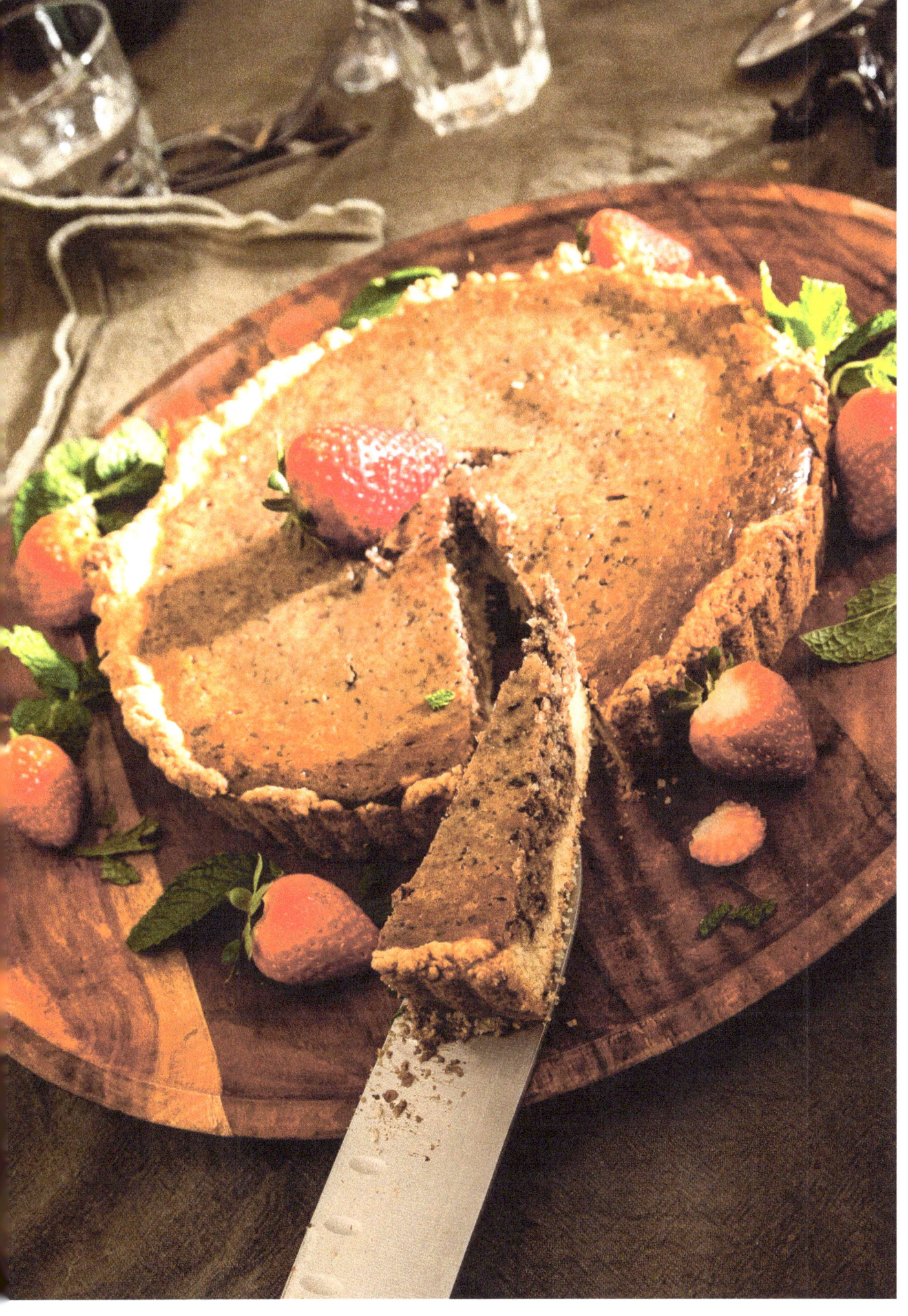

Chocolate, Orange and Lavender Soft Centre Pudding

MAKES 6

1 orange

6 teaspoons marmalade

1 teaspoon dried culinary lavender

200 grams dark chocolate

150 grams butter

1/3 cup brown sugar

¼ cup caster sugar

4 eggs

¼ cup plain flour

Preheat your oven to 180°C. Grease 6 small ramekins and set them on a baking tray.

In a small saucepan or a bowl over simmering water, gently melt together the dark chocolate, butter, both sugars, zest from the orange and lavender. Stir until smooth and glossy, then remove from the heat and let cool slightly. Beat in the eggs and fold through flour. Fold in the segments from the orange.

Spoon half the mixture into the base of each ramekin. Add a small teaspoon-sized blob of marmalade into the centre of each, then cover with the remaining chocolate mixture.

Bake for about 20 minutes, until the tops are set but the centres are still soft. Let them rest a minute before serving.

Serve warm with thick cream or vanilla ice-cream.

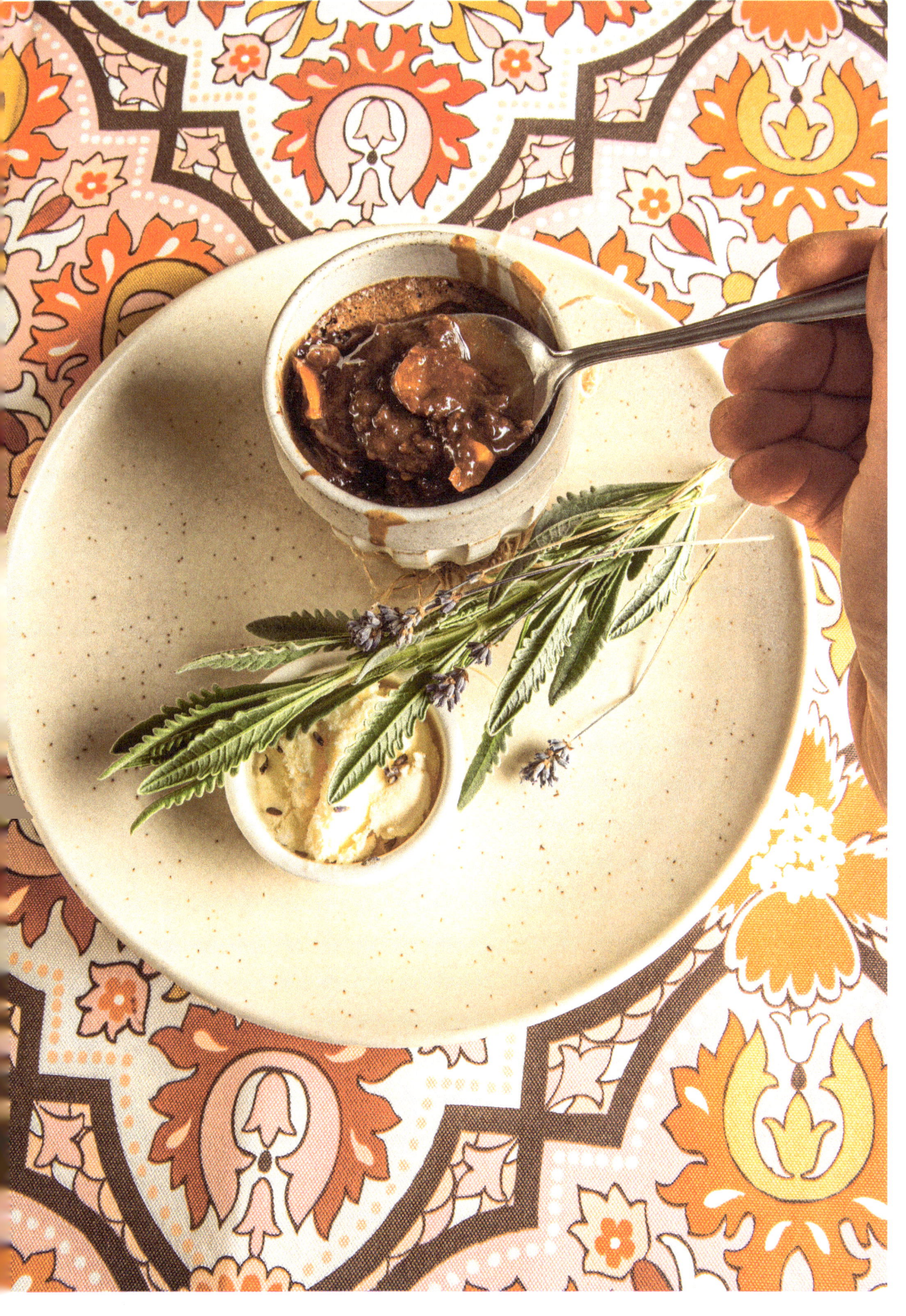

Lavender Infused Panna Cotta

MAKES 6

2 cups pouring cream

1 cup full cream milk

½ teaspoon dried culinary lavender

1 vanilla bean, split (or 1 tsp vanilla paste)

1/3 cup caster sugar

2½ teaspoons powdered gelatine

2 tablespoons hot water

Place the cream, milk, lavender, vanilla and sugar in a saucepan. Gently heat until just below a simmer—do not boil. Let it infuse off the heat for 10–15 minutes, then strain to remove the lavender and vanilla pod, or leave in the lavender if you want the flavour to intensify.

Meanwhile, sprinkle the gelatine over the water in a small bowl and let it disolve. Stir the gelatine into the warm cream mixture until completely dissolved. strain if needed

Pour into lightly oiled moulds, ramekins or glasses. Chill until set—at least 4 hours or overnight.

Serve cold, turned out or in their vessels, with a generous handful of fresh berries. Raspberries, blueberries, blackberries, or sliced strawberries all work beautifully and coulis or syrup.

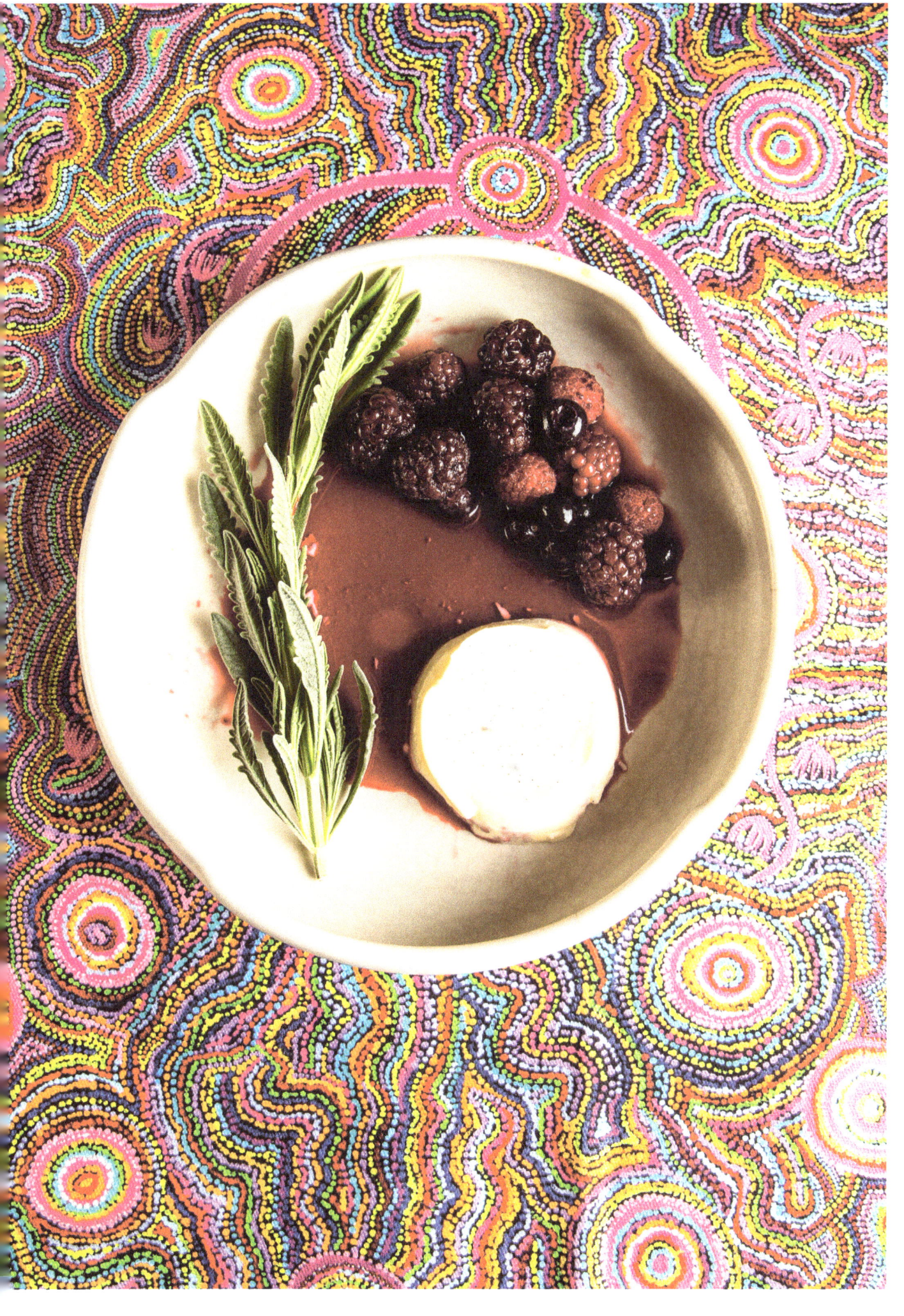

Pork Crumbed with Sage, Garlic and Lavender

SERVES 4

4 pork loin chops, cutlets or steaks

sea salt and cracked pepper

few tablespoons plain flour

2 eggs

½ cup milk

1 cup fresh or panko breadcrumbs

2 teaspoons dried culinary lavender

1 tablespoon fresh sage

2 cloves garlic

1 lemon

splash olive oil

a knob of butter

Set up three bowls for crumbing—one with flour, one with the beaten eggs mixed with the mik, and one with the breadcrumbs.

To the breadcrumbs, add the lavender, sage, chopped garlic, salt and pepper, lemon zest and parmesan. Stir together with your hands or a fork so the flavours are well mixed through.

Dip each pork cutlet first in the flour, shaking off any excess, then into the egg, and finally press into the breadcrumb mixture. Make sure each piece is well coated.

Heat a generous splash of olive oil in a large frying pan over medium heat. Add a knob of butter. Cook the pork gently on each side over a low heat until golden and cooked through.

Lovely with apple and fennel slaw, mustardy mash, or just lemon wedges and a bitter green salad.

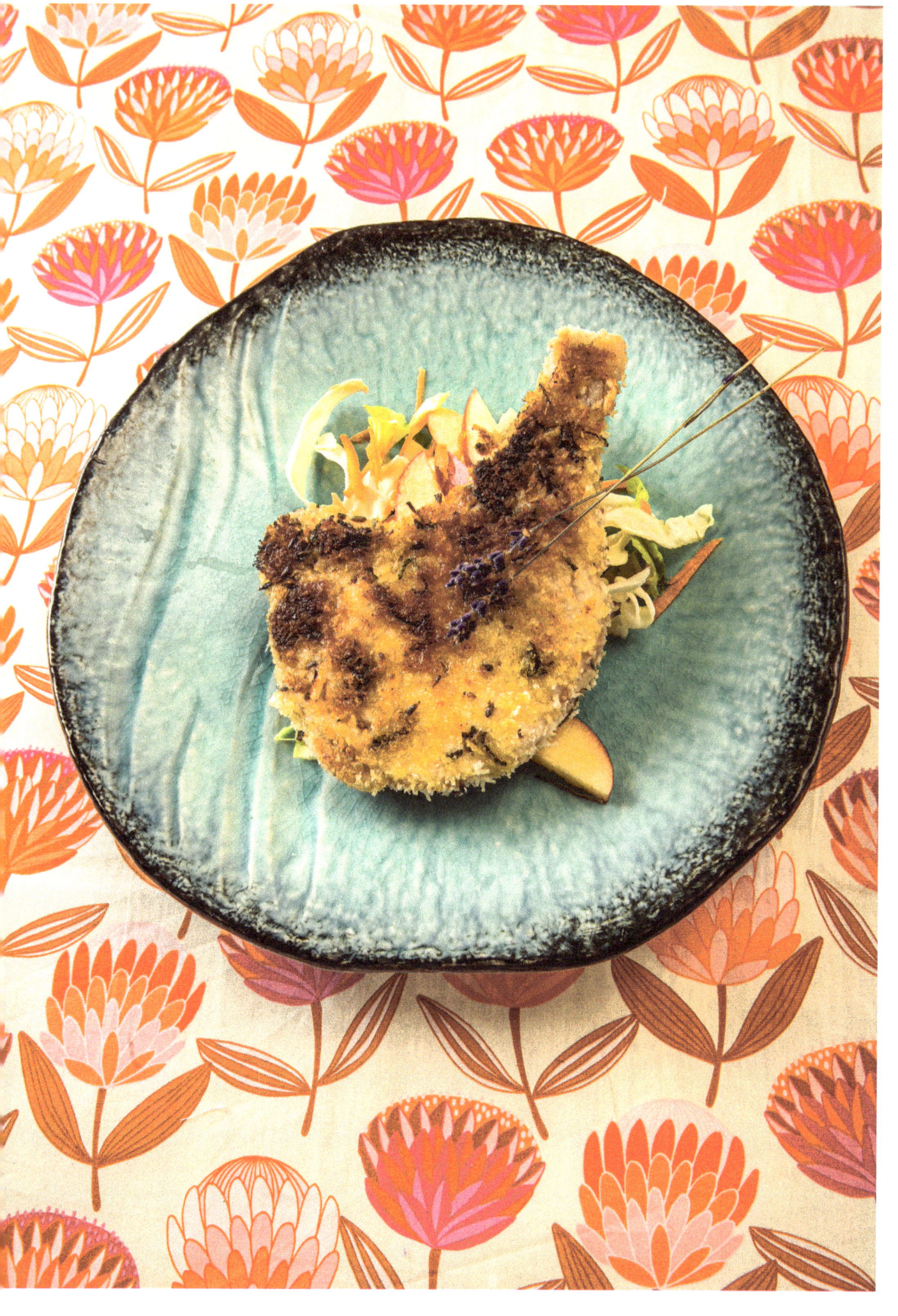

White Chocolate Eclairs with Lavender and Raspberry

MAKES 8 LARGE

CHOUX PASTRY

100 grams unsalted butter

1 cup water

pinch of salt

1 cup plain flour

4 free-range eggs

LAVENDER AND RASPBERRY CUSTARD

2 cups full cream milk

1 teaspoon dried culinary lavender

1 teaspoon vanilla bean paste

4 egg yolks

1/3 cup caster sugar

¼ cup cornflour

1 tablespoon unsalted butter

½ cup fresh or frozen raspberries (plus extra for garnish)

WHITE CHOCOLATE GLAZE

200 grams white chocolate

1/4 cup cream

Turn the oven onto 200°C. To make the choux pastry, bring the butter, water and salt to the boil in a saucepan. Add the flour all at once and stir quickly with a wooden spoon until the mixture comes together and pulls away from the sides. Continue stirring over low heat for a minute or two to dry it out slightly.

Transfer to a bowl and allow to cool slightly. Beat in the eggs one at a time, mixing well between each, until the dough is glossy and holds its shape when piped.

Spoon or pipe onto a lined baking tray in éclair shapes, leaving space between each. Bake in a hot oven at 200°C until puffed, golden and crisp. Cool completely on a wire rack.

To make the custard, gently warm the milk in a saucepan with the lavender and vanilla until just below simmering. Take off the heat and allow the lavender to steep for about ten minutes. Strain out the lavender (or leave it in for a more intense taste).

In a separate bowl, whisk the egg yolks, sugar, and cornflour until pale. Slowly pour the warm milk into the egg mixture, whisking constantly. Return the mixture to the pan and stir over medium heat until thick and smooth. Remove from heat and stir in the butter. Fold through the raspberries while the custard is still warm, gently crushing a few to ripple the colour.

Spoon into a bowl or piping bag, cover with baking paper or cling film directly on the surface to prevent it forming a thick skin and chill in the fridge until firm.

For the glaze, gently melt the chocolate and cream together in a bowl over a pot of simmering water. Dip the tops of each éclair into the glaze.

To fill, slice each éclair through the side or base and pipe in the lavender raspberry crème pâtissière.

Best enjoyed the day they're made.

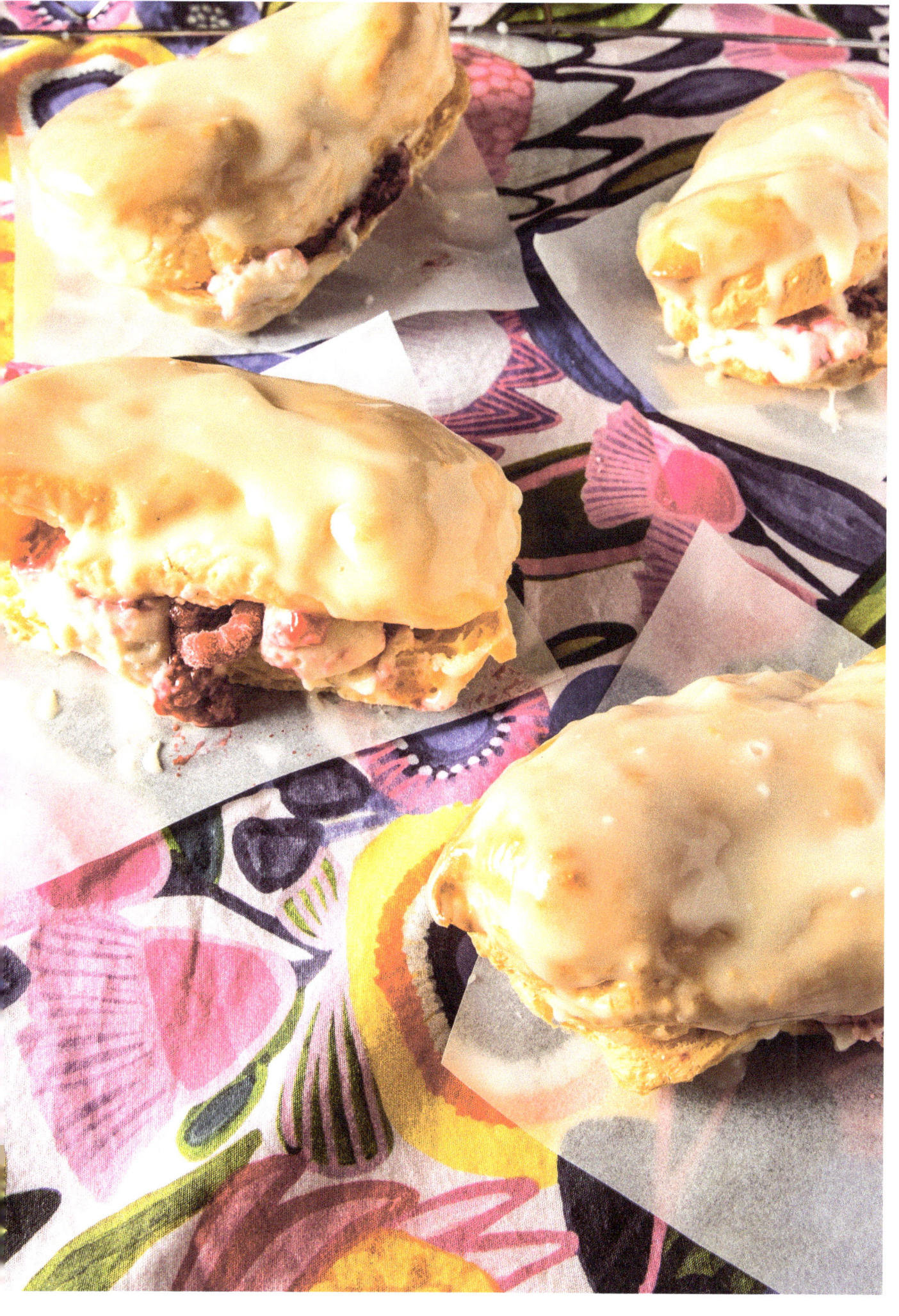

Lavender Honey Ice-cream or Parfait

SERVES 8

If you have the equpiment to churn the icecream do that. Otherwise freeze it in a pan loaf and slice with some syrup to serve as a parfait.

2 cups pure cream
1 cup full cream milk
½ cup good quality honey
1 tablespoon dried culinary lavender
5 egg yolks
pinch of sea salt

Warm the cream, milk and honey gently in a saucepan with the lavender. Bring just to a simmer, then turn off the heat and let it steep for fifteen to twenty minutes. Strain out the lavender if you prefer and return the infused cream to the pan. Or leave the lavender in for a more instense flavour.

In a separate bowl, whisk the egg yolks with a pinch of salt until smooth and slightly thickened. Slowly pour the warm cream into the yolks, whisking constantly. Return the mixture to the saucepan and cook over low heat, stirring with a wooden spoon or spatula, until it thickens slightly and coats the back of the spoon—don't let it boil.

Strain the custard into a clean bowl. Chill completely in the fridge, ideally overnight, for the best flavour and texture.

Churn in an ice cream maker until softly set, then freeze until firm. If you don't have a machine, pour into a shallow tray, freeze until starting to firm, then stir well with a fork or blend and return to the freezer. Repeat a few times for a smoother result. Or just let it set hard and slice for a parfait.

Serve on its own, with stewed rhubarb or roasted apricots, or sandwiched between lavender shortbread for something special.

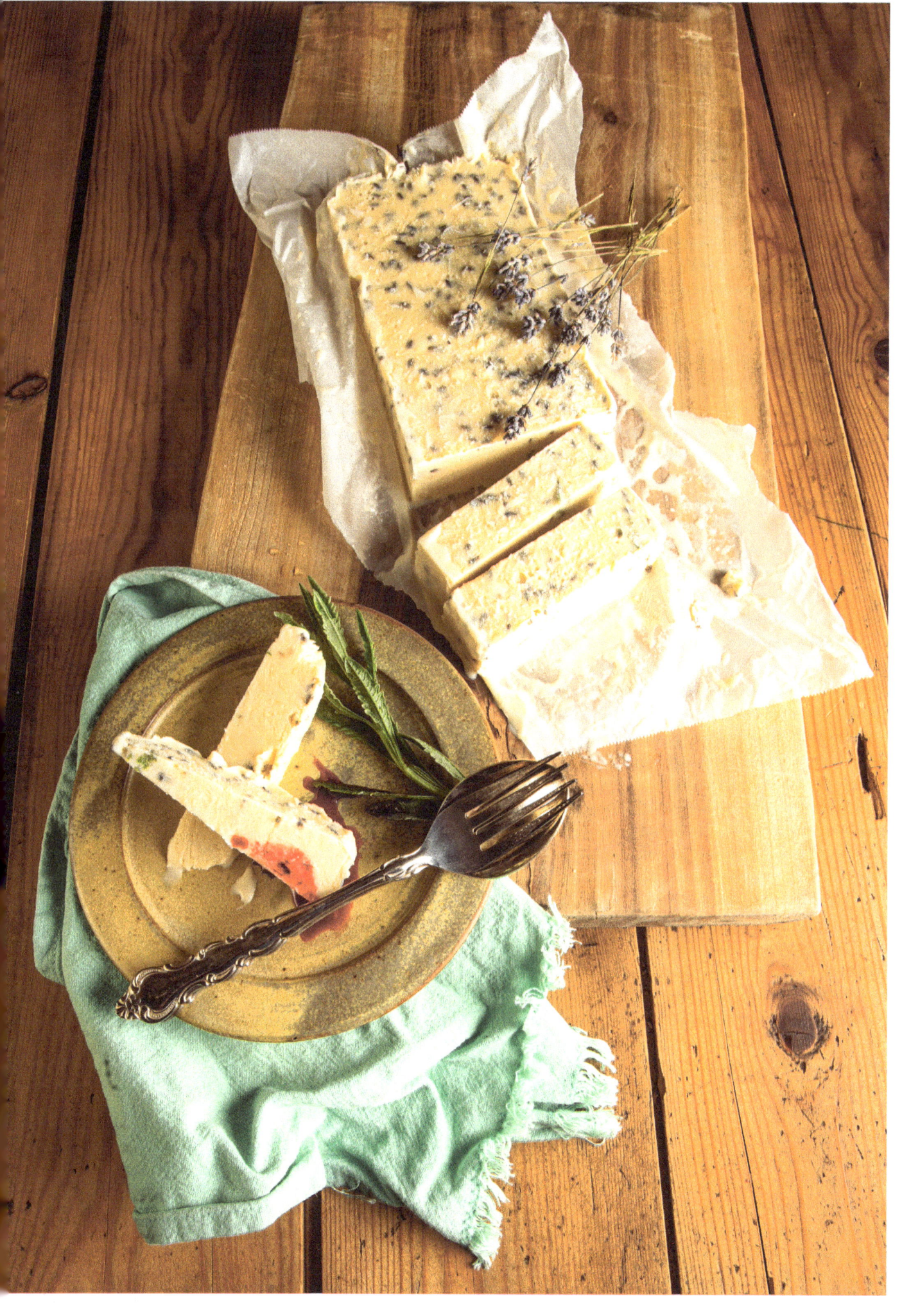

Indulgent Lavender Hot Chocolate

MAKES 2

2 cups full cream milk

100g good-quality dark chocolate

1 teaspoon dried culinary lavender

½ teaspoon ground cinnamon

1 teaspoon honey or raw sugar

pinch of sea salt

Gently heat the milk in a small saucepan with the lavender, cinnamon and a small pinch of salt. Bring just to a simmer, then remove from the heat and let the flavours steep for five to ten minutes.

Strain out the lavender, return the milk to the pan and add the chopped chocolate. Stir gently over low heat until the chocolate is fully melted and the drink is smooth and glossy. Sweeten to taste with a little honey or sugar, if desired.

Froth with a stick blender or whisk if you like it velvety.

Pour into warm mugs and serve as is, or top with softly whipped cream and a few lavender buds for a little flourish.

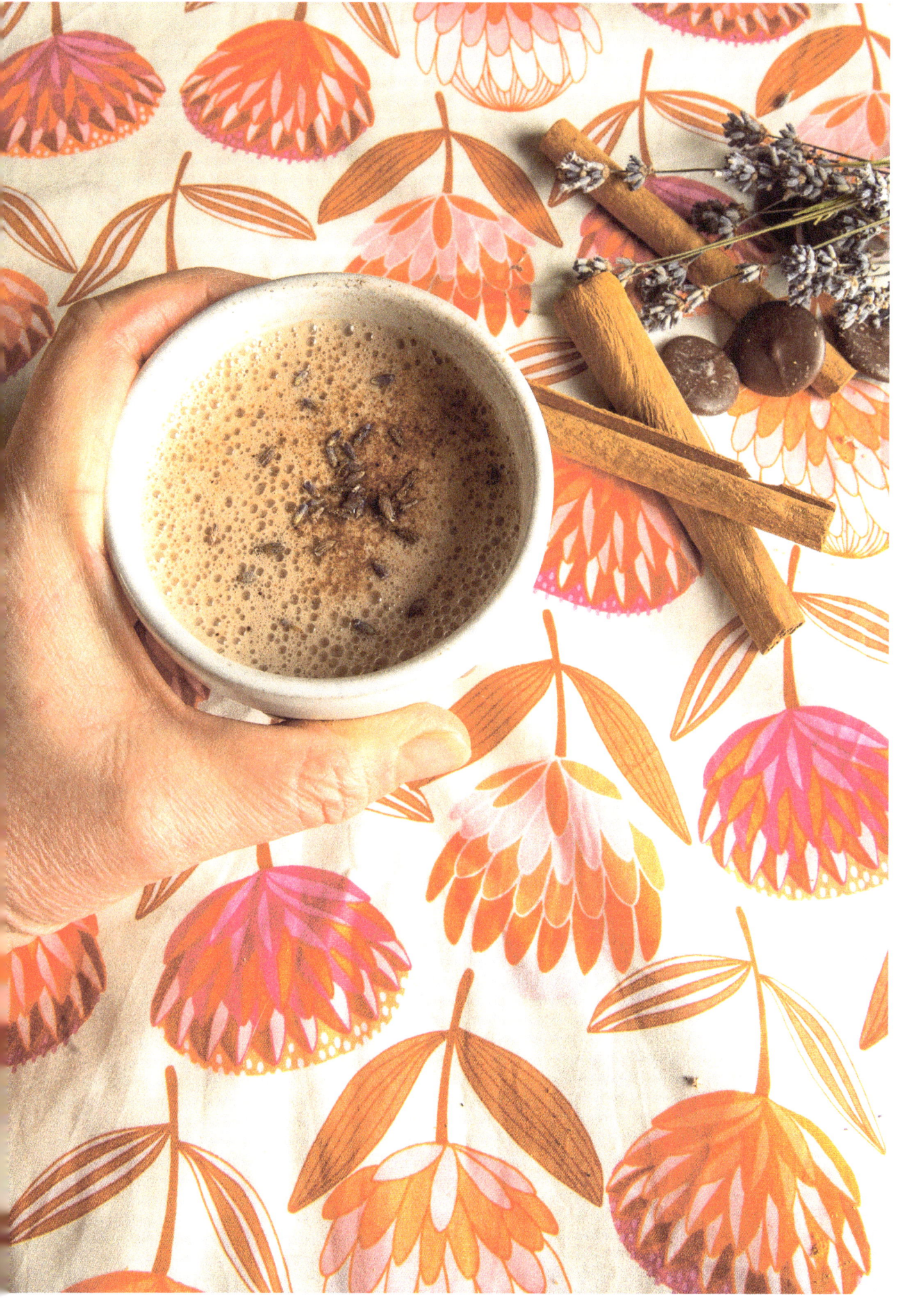

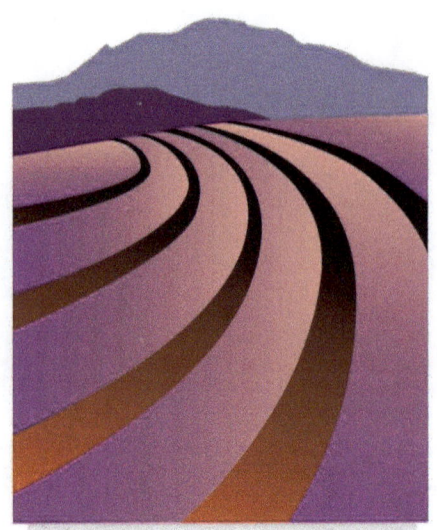

BRIDESTOWE LAVENDER ESTATE
Made in Tasmania, loved worldwide

Located in Nabowla, Tasmania, Bridestowe Lavender Estate is a celebrated lavender farm crafting premium products that embody the region's pristine beauty. Their aromatic range includes essential oils, skincare, and culinary items, reflecting Tasmania's unique terroir. With vibrant fields and sustainable practices, Bridestowe blends tradition and innovation. Visitors can explore the scenic estate, enjoy lavender-infused treats at the café, or shop for quality gifts. Committed to eco-friendly methods, Bridestowe delivers a sensory experience of relaxation and craftsmanship. Discover the timeless allure of lavender with their exceptional offerings.

03 6352 8182
296 Gillespies Rd, Nabowla, TAS 7260
info@bridestowelavender.com.au
www.bridestowelavender.com.au

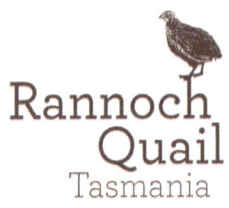

RANNOCH QUAIL TASMANIA

Premium quail from Coal River Valley, offering butterfly boned, whole, hot smoked quail & eggs. With over 30 years of eco-friendly practices, this 100% Tasmanian family-owned business delivers nature's finest flavors.

0484 002 519 | admin@rannochquail.com.au
www.rannochquail.com.au

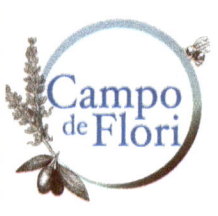

CAMPO DE FLORI

Tasmania's unique farm with lavender fields, olive grove, and bee apiary. Award-winning saffron and culinary lavender, plus lavender tea, honey, olive oil, and artisan pottery. Available at Salamanca Market and select retailers.

0409643256 | lisa@campodeflori.com.au
www.campodeflori.com

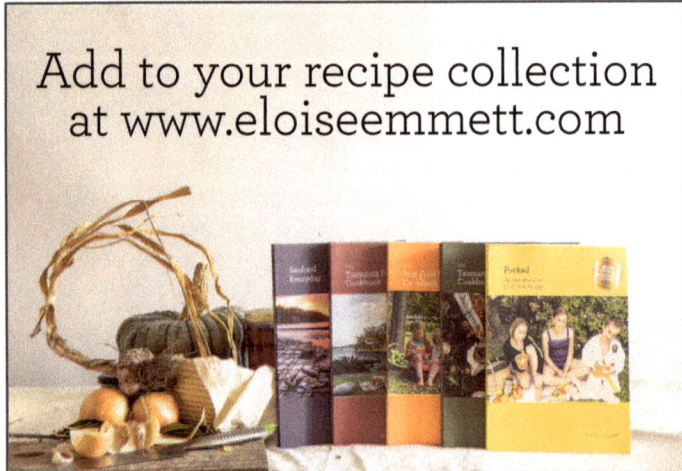

Add to your recipe collection at www.eloiseemmett.com

TASMANIAN LAVENDER COMPANY

Premium lavender products crafted in Port Arthur, Tasmania. Committed to quality, their offerings capture the region's natural beauty and fragrance.

(03) 6250 3058 | info@portarthurlavender.com.au
www.portarthurlavender.com.au

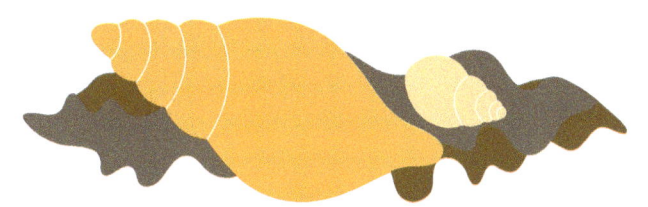

TERALINA BEACH HOUSE

Premium Family Accommodation

stay@teralinabeachhouse.com
www.teralinabeachhouse.com

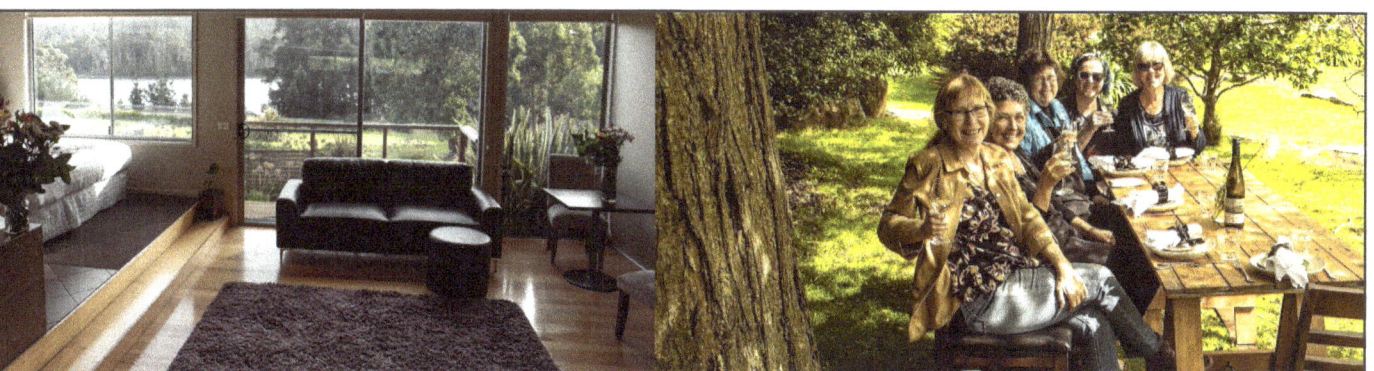

Little Norfolk Bay
BISTRO & CHALETS

Bistro, Accommodation, Cooking Retreats & Workshops in Taranna on the gorgeous Tasman Peninsula. Perfect for corporate or private gatherings and celebrations.

www.littlenorfolkbaybistroandchalets.com

About the Author

Eloise Emmett is a Trade Qualified Chef with over 30 years experience in commercial kitchens, including 7 years as the Chef and owner of her own popular restaurant The Mussel Boys on the Tasman Peninsula. She now runs a Bistro with accomdation and a boutique cooking school that hosts cooking workshops and weekend cooking retreats, Little Norfolk Bay Bistro and Chalets. Eloise has been writing and photographing recipes for her popular website eloiseemmett.com since 2012. In 2013, Eloise co-authored the *Bream Creek Farmers Market Cookbook*. In 2015 she published *The Real Food for Kids Cookbook* and in 2016 she published the multi award winning *Seafood Everyday*. *Seafood Everyday* won **Best Fish and Seafood Book in Australia**, and **Best Book by a Woman Chef in Australia**. It then went on to become the third best seafood cookbook in the world, when it and won third place in **The Best Fish and Seafood** category at the **Gourmand World Cookbook Awards**. In 2017 Eloise published the first print of *The Tasmania Pantry* and in 2020 she published the second edition, *The Tasmania Pantry 2*. Both books won national Gourmand Cookbook awards. She then went on to publish "Packed' and "Celebrate" in 2022. This is her 7th solo book but she has helped many others self publish and has contributed to many cookbooks over the years.

Eloise loves cooking, styling and photographing food and shopping for props at op-shops and markets. She has three children with her fisherman husband and they live on the stunning Tasman Peninsula in Tasmania. Most of all Eloise, loves educating families about how important cooking, preparing meals and eating real food is. Her core message, is that cooking is not hard and is a lot more economical way to feed your family and she encourages even the bussiest families to prepare easy meals from real food.

www.eloiseemmett.com

Outro

Thanks for purchasing this book and supporting my small business. Thank you to the people involved in the production of this book, the designer Kylie Berry Design and The Art of Words Studio, my editors daughter Maggie Emmett and mum Bernadette. There are only a few of us involved in the production of this book, unlike a published book that has a big budget and many staff involved. Although I have edited until my eyes go blurry about 200 times and I am not that great at sitting still in front of a computer at the best of times, I am sure there will be the odd mistake or two. Let's hope they are little grammatical typos and not addition cups of chillies or something hideous like that! Please let me know if you see anything so I can fix for future print runs. Email me at eloiseemmett@gmail.com. Hopefully you can see them as little quirks in this handmade product, that is totally produced in Tasmania

Recipes, photography and words © Eloise Emmett

Design © Kylie Berry

No part of this book can be copied without permission, includes photocopying and photos of the pages.

Although I have researched the dietary information and other info carefully (for about 30 years!!) it is still only my opinion, so please always talk to a health professional. I will not be liable for any injuries or damage as a result of following the information and recipes in this book.

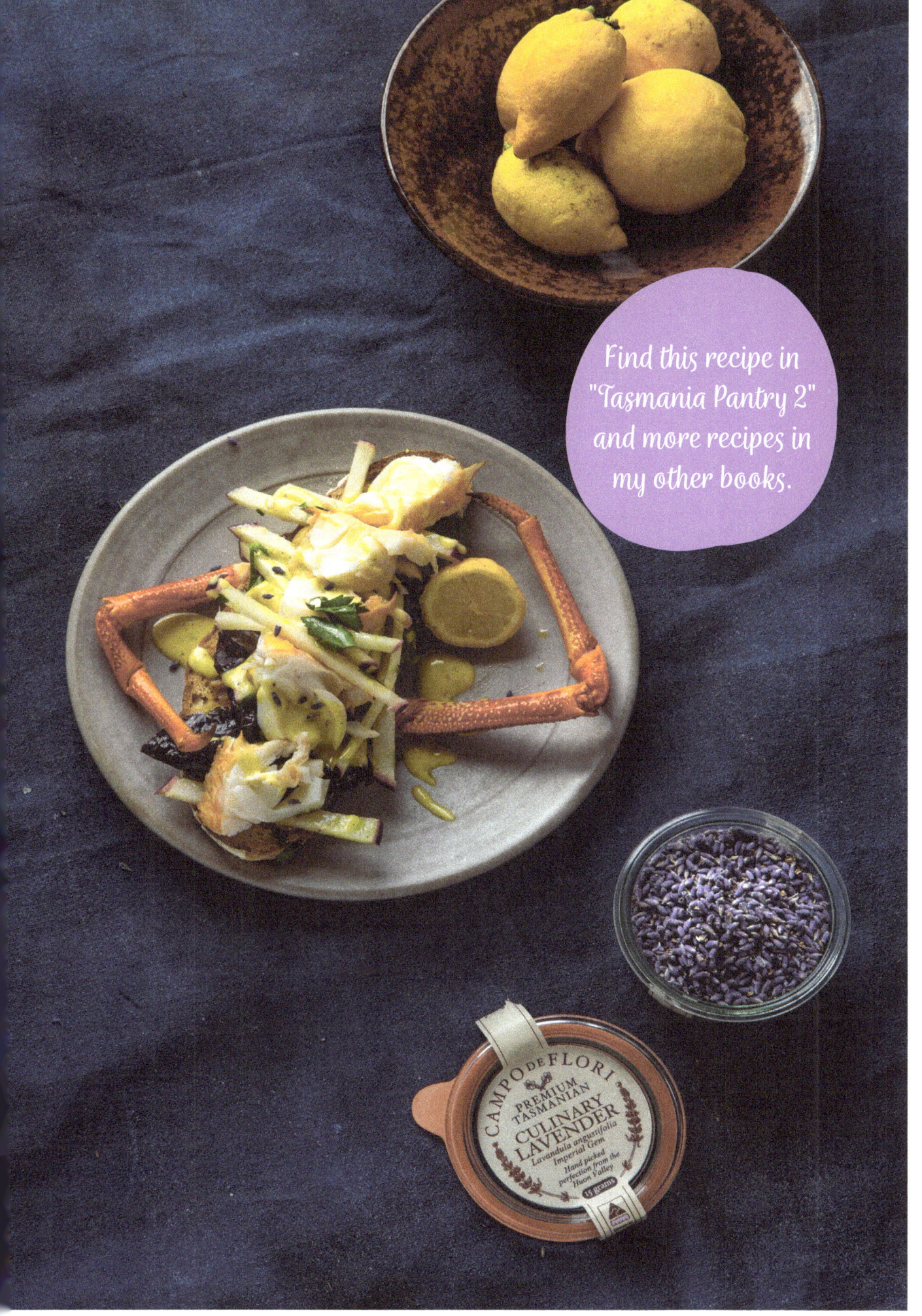

Find this recipe in "Tasmania Pantry 2" and more recipes in my other books.

INDEX

Apple and Lavender Crumble 62

Apple, Cinnamon, Honey and
Lavender Tea Cake 54

Blackberry Lavender Syrup 68

Burnt Butter, Rosemary, Lavender
and Honey Cake 66

Buttermilk Fried Rannoch Quail 12

Chicken in French Mustard and Lavender Sauce 38

Chicken with Quince and Lavender 76

Chocolate, Orange and Lavender Soft Centre
Pudding 80

Chocolate Ricotta and Lavender Pie 78

Creme Brulee with Lavender and Raspberry 70

Duck Breast with Blueberry and Lavender Sauce 32

Duck with Mulberry and Lavender Relish
and Apple Slaw 14

Foccacia with Herbs de Provence 58

Goats Cheese and Lavender Beetroot Tart 22

Granola with Lavender and Honey 60

Grilled Octopus with Honey, Oregano, Lemon,
Lavender and Garlic Marinade 48

Honey and Lavender Dressed Apricot Chicken
Summer Garden Salad 52

Indulgent Lavender Hot Chocolate 90

Lavender and Blueberry Pancakes 16

Lavender Custard Tart with Fruit 50

Lavender Honey Icecream/parfait 88

Lavender Infused Pannacotta 82

Lavender Mayonaise Prawn Cocktail 34

Mackeral Baked with Lemon, Olive Oil,
Lavender and Bush Herbs 74

Pan-Fried Boarfish with Lavender
and Blueberry Butter Sauce 46

Pork Belly with Plum and Lavender 24

Pork Crumbed with Sage, Garlic and Lavender 84

Pork Loin with Honey, Mustard
and Lavender Sauce 72

Porterhouse with Prawns in a Garlic and
Herbs de Provence Sauce 30

Potato, Leek and Ham Soup
with Herbs de Provence 10

Rosemary, Garlic and Lavender Pull Apart Bread 20

Slow Cooked Beef with Apple, Dijon, Lavender
and Native Pepper 40

Slow Cooked Mediterranean Lamb Shoulder 44

Smoked Fish Pate 42

Sour Cherry, Verjuice and Lavender Jelly,
Honey Custard Trifle 26

Steamed Parrot Fish, Dijon, Lemon, Mandarin
and Lavender 64

Venison Fillet Marinated with Pepperberry,
Lavender Leaf and Rosemary
with Spiced Quinces 28

Watermelon Lavender Bubbly Cocktail 36

White Chocolate, Blueberry and Lavender
Baked Cheesecake 56

White Chocolate Eclairs with Lavender and
Raspberry 86

White Chocolate Lavender Cookies 18